A VIDEO ATLAS OF NEUROMUSCULAR DISORDERS

A VIDEO ATLAS OF NEUROMUSCULAR DISORDERS

Aziz Shaibani, MD, FACP, FAAN

DIRECTOR, NERVE AND MUSCLE CENTER OF TEXAS, HOUSTON, TEXAS
CLINICAL PROFESSOR OF MEDICINE, BAYLOR COLLEGE OF MEDICINE
ADJUNCT PROFESSOR OF NEUROLOGY, KANSAS UNIVERSITY
MEDICAL CENTER

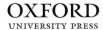

OXFORD
UNIVERSITY PRESS

Oxford University Press is a department of the University of
Oxford. It furthers the University's objective of excellence in research,
scholarship, and education by publishing worldwide.

Oxford   New York
Auckland   Cape Town   Dar es Salaam   Hong Kong   Karachi
Kuala Lumpur   Madrid   Melbourne   Mexico City   Nairobi
New Delhi   Shanghai   Taipei   Toronto

With offices in
Argentina   Austria   Brazil   Chile   Czech Republic   France   Greece
Guatemala   Hungary   Italy   Japan   Poland   Portugal   Singapore
South Korea   Switzerland   Thailand   Turkey   Ukraine   Vietnam

Oxford is a registered trademark of Oxford University Press
in the UK and certain other countries.

Published in the United States of America by
Oxford University Press
198 Madison Avenue, New York, NY 10016

Library of Congress Cataloging-in-Publication Data
Shaibani, Aziz, author.
A video atlas of neuromuscular disorders / Aziz Shaibani.
     p. ; cm.
Includes bibliographical references.
ISBN 978–0–19–989815–2 (alk. paper)
I. Title.
[DNLM: 1. Neuromuscular Diseases—physiopathology—Atlases.   2. Neuromuscular Diseases—
physiopathology—Case Reports.   3. Neurologic Manifestations—Atlases.   4. Neurologic Manifestations—
Case Reports. WE 17]
RC925.55
616.7′44—dc23
2014003753ss

The science of medicine is a rapidly changing field. As new research and clinical experience broaden our knowledge,
changes in treatment and drug therapy occur. The author and publisher of this work have checked with sources believed
to be reliable in their efforts to provide information that is accurate and complete, and in accordance with the standards
accepted at the time of publication. However, in light of the possibility of human error or changes in the practice
of medicine, neither the author, nor the publisher, nor any other party who has been involved in the preparation or
publication of this work warrants that the information contained herein is in every respect accurate or complete. Readers
are encouraged to confirm the information contained herein with other reliable sources, and are strongly advised to check
the product information sheet provided by the pharmaceutical company for each drug they plan to administer.

9 8 7 6 5 4 3 2 1
Printed in the United States of America
on acid-free paper

CONTENTS

FOREWORD

I t is a pleasure to write a foreword for Dr. Aziz Shaibani's *Video Atlas of Neuromuscular Disorders*. Why do we need another book on neuromuscular disease? We currently have several successful textbooks in the market that cover muscle and nerve disorders. The answer is that Dr. Shaibani has put together a truly unique volume that fills a niche not currently covered. His book provides a large number of outstanding videos of patients who exhibit signs of neuromuscular problems that we all encounter in our clinics.

Dr. Shaibani is uniquely qualified to author such a scholarly contribution. Dr. Shaibani completed his neurology residency and neuromuscular fellowship at the Baylor School of Medicine. He immediately established a premier neuromuscular practice in the center of the largest medical center in the world, Texas Medical Center. Despite the fact that there were neuromuscular programs at several universities in Houston, Dr. Shaibani's practice has thrived and continues to expand. This, of course, is because Dr. Shaibani is a master clinician in the field of neuromuscular disease, and patients come to him from throughout the United States as well as internationally for his expert opinion and care. He continues to be closely affiliated with the academic neurology and internal medicine programs in the University of Texas and Baylor College of Medicine.

In addition, we have developed extremely close ties with Dr. Shaibani at our own University of Kansas Medical Center, where he holds a position of adjunct professor of neurology, because of our many collaborative academic and research projects. Dr. Shaibani is an active member of important national neuromuscular organizations such as the Muscle Study Group and the Western ALS Study Group. He has been an investigator in dozens of important neuromuscular research clinical trials.

But back to this video atlas. Clearly Professor Shaibani has accomplished what many of us have hoped we would do in our busy neuromuscular practices. He has taken the time and effort to meticulously video record the patients he sees in his practice if they exhibit any typical or even atypical neurology signs as a manifestation of their disorder. It is clear watching these videos that they are done in real time, in the office, and without sophisticated equipment. In this way, he has managed to give us multiple examples of a disease manifestation such as myotonia, its variants, or facioscapulohumeral muscular dystrophy, in its various forms, as some of the many, many examples. It should be noted that all patients have given written permission for Dr. Shaibani to use these videos for publication.

I've also realized there is some degree of variability as well as some degree of consistency in the manifestations of neuromuscular disease that we observe in patients. What Professor Shaibani has done is amazing in that he has recorded multiple presentations of these neurologic signs for us to compare and examine. The video atlas is organized in chapters of the various neuromuscular disorders. Each series of videos has an accompanying brief, well-written summary of the disease and the various signs that will be demonstrated on the videos. Accurate and usable references are supplied.

This video atlas, I am sure, will become popular with a wide range of learners. Of course, neurology residents and neuromuscular fellows, clinical neurophysiology fellows, and junior faculty and practitioners of neuromuscular medicine will clearly benefit by seeing multiple examples of neuromuscular clinical signs. I believe that early learners, such as undergraduates, medical students, and perhaps research PhDs will benefit by being able to see these examples for perhaps the first and only time in their careers. Finally, I do believe that experienced neuromuscular practitioners, such as myself and my many colleagues, will find great value in having these videos as a resource for teaching various learners. I think we will all be a bit envious that we did not take the time and effort to collect videos so extensively in this fashion.

So, I would like to give a huge "congratulations" to Dr. Aziz Shaibani for his remarkable efforts in putting together this *Video Atlas of Neuromuscular Disorders*. I know from many conversations with Aziz that this was a true labor of love that took him many years to create. We in the neuromuscular community are most appreciative of Dr. Shaibani for having provided us with this unique academic contribution to our field. I hope Aziz keeps recording videos in his practice and that future editions will be forthcoming with time. I know this atlas will be a great success.

Richard J. Barohn, MD
Gertrude and Dewey Ziegler Professor and Chair, Department of Neurology
University Distinguished Professor
University of Kansas Medical Center
Kansas City, Kansas

FOREWORD

It is truly an honor for me to write the foreword for this neuromuscular video atlas edited by Dr. Aziz Shaibani. Dr. Shaibani is the Director of the Nerve and Muscle Center of Texas and a Clinical Professor of Medicine at Baylor College of Medicine and Adjunct Professor of Neurology at the University of Kansas. I've known Dr. Shaibani for two decades, since I too was in Texas. He has an extensive experience evaluating and treating patients with neuromuscular diseases and in training medical students, residents, and fellows. Over the years, he has videotaped patient examinations and has created a catalog of rare and common neurological signs in patients with a wide range of neuromuscular disorders.

In this atlas, Dr. Shaibani presents 280 of these video cases. The videos include patients describing their symptoms and pertinent neuromuscular examination. Each video is accompanied by a clinical synopsis of the case, and in some cases EMG videos and figures of biopsies. Each case is followed by a question and answer for the viewers (e.g., guess the next test, correct diagnosis, or treatment), a discussion, and references. As is apparent in this video atlas, Dr. Shaibani is an astute clinician and an excellent teacher. It is one thing to read about various neuromuscular signs and disorders in textbooks, but another to actually see them. Thus, I enthusiastically recommend this video atlas for neurologists and physiatrists who evaluate patients with neuromuscular conditions. I congratulate Dr. Shaibani for his valuable contribution to the field.

Anthony Amato, MD
Vice Chairman
Department of Neurology
Chief, Neuromuscular Division
Brigham and Women's Hospital
Professor of Neurology
Harvard Medical School
Boston, Massachusetts

PREFACE

The idea for this atlas is derived from an appreciation for the need of a new method of learning in the age of electronic communications and reduced attention span. Instead of spending time to reconstruct mental images of complicated neuromuscular cases from a lengthy and often dry text, this video atlas will allow viewers to spend that time to figure out the diagnostic and therapeutic challenges of these cases—an intellectual process that is intended to enforce clinical skills, which are invaluable for the profession of medicine.

Two hundred sixty-four video cases are artistically produced to express the manifestations of different neuromuscular diseases. Each case is described and is followed by one or multiple-choice questions. One page is dedicated to highlight salient points about the topic and to provide an update for the experts.

The book is divided into 28 chapters, each containing several cases. The chapters are not related to each other, and they can be read separately according to the interest of the reader. Each case is separately "clickable" from the index of cases at the beginning of each chapter. The material reflects information about common and rare neuromuscular disorders such as myasthenia gravis, amyotrophic lateral sclerosis (ALS), muscular dystrophy, chronic inflammatory demyelinating polyneuropathy (CIDP), stiff person syndrome (SPS), myopathies, and neuropathies.

The description and multiple choice questions (MCQs) make the book ideal for medical students, neurology residents, and subspecialty fellows who are preparing for their board examinations, while the updates are more suited to address issues at the level of neuromuscular specialists and practicing neurologists.

This book is by no means a textbook in neuromuscular disorders, but rather a "sharpener" of neuromuscular skills and decision-making for those who already have acquired the basic necessary medical knowledge.

A book is, after all, a personal experience. The text material of this book reflects our experience and knowledge in neuromuscular medicine. I have chosen to emphasize certain aspects of neuromuscular medicine and ignore others, depending on my appreciation of their significance. Whenever references are used, they have been cited after each case. I also relied on two major resources: *Neuromuscular Disorders* by Anthony Amato and James Russell and the website of the neuromuscular disease center at Washington University (http://neuromuscular. wustl.edu/).

Aziz Shaibani, M.D.

ACKNOWLEDGMENT

I would like to profusely thank the following colleagues for their critical review of cases from the atlas: Sendra Ajroud-Driss, M.D., Brent Beson, M.D., David Gehret, M.D., Melanie Doerflinger Glenn, M.D., James Howard, M.D., Viktoriya Irodenko, M.D., Liberty Jenkin, M.D., Vikas Kumar, M.D., Todd Levine, M D., Teerin Liewluck, M.D., Jau-Shin Lou, M.D., Blanca Marky, M.D., Matt Mayer, M.D., Tahseen Mozaffar, M.D., Sabrina Paganoni, M.D., Michael Pulley, M.D., Devon Rubin, M.D., David Saperstein, M.D., Sona Shah, M.D., Maryam Tahmasbi Sohi, M.D., Rabie Tawil, M.D., Steven Vernino, M.D., and the rest of Rick's real neuromuscular friends (www.rrnmf.com).

Special thanks go to Duaa Jabari, M.D., and Nawar Hussin, M.D., for their technical support and to Randolph Evans, M.D., for encouragement and review.

I would like to thank the referring physicians for their confidence in our center, and I thank the patients, the primary source of information, for allowing us to publish their videos for educational purposes.

Finally, the time to prepare this work was taken away from family time, and I would like to thank my wife Arwa and our children, Ahmad, Senan, and Rami, for allowing me to do so.

Aziz Shaibani, M.D.

GAIT DISORDERS

CASE 1.1: BILATERAL FOOT DROP

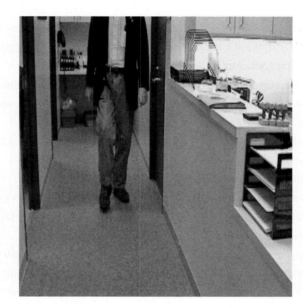

VIDEO 1.1

A 67-year-old man presented with a 3-year history of gradually worsening gait imbalance, feet numbness, and hand grip weakness. Gait is shown in the video. Examination also showed moderate impairment of sensation to vibration and proprioception in the feet and diffuse areflexia. Proximal strength was normal. Nerve conduction study (NCS) revealed that distal motor latencies of the bilateral peroneal and tibial nerves were 9–11 msec with mild asymmetry. Their median and ulnar counterparts were 6–7 msec. Compound muscle action potential (CMAP) amplitudes were preserved and the sural responses were absent. F waves were mildly prolonged. Cerebrospinal fluid (CSF) protein was 110 mg/dl. Immunoglobin G (IgG) synthesis rate was increased. Immunofixation protein electrophoresis (IFPE) revealed immunoglobin M (IgM) lambda spike.

The diagnosis would be supported by an abnormal:

1. Myelin-associated glycoprotein (MAG) antibody titer
2. Sulfatide antibody titer
3. Charcot-Marie-Tooth (CMT) mutation analysis
4. Blood lead level
5. Porphyrins in the urine

DIAGNOSIS

- Video gait analysis: weak ankle dorsiflexion results in decreased toe clearance and foot "slap" during heel strike. Compensation often occurs through excessive hip flexion during the swing phase, referred to as a steppage gait pattern.
- Foot drop may result from any insult at the level of the deep peroneal nerve, common peroneal nerve, sciatic nerve, lumbosacral (LS) plexus, nerve roots, motor neurons, neuromuscular junction (NMJ), muscles, spinal cord, and brain.
- Preservation of the ankle invertors is against L5 radiculopathy and is in favor of peroneal neuropathy since ankle invertors are tibially innervated.
- Painful asymmetrical foot drop is typically seen in vasculitis.
- Painless asymmetrical foot drop with preserved ankle reflexes is typically seen in amyotrophic lateral sclerosis (ALS), myasthenia gravis (MG), and distal myopathies. Foot drop may be the first presenting feature of ALS.
- Chronic inflammatory demyelinating polyneuropathy (CIDP) patients may present with foot drop, especially the distal acquired demyelinating sensorimotor neuropathy (DADSAM), which is associated with MAG antibodies and is refractory to treatment.
- Facioscapulohumeral muscular dystrophy (FSHD) may present with foot drop. Preservation or hypertrophy of the extensor digitorum brevis (EDB) muscle distinguishes myopathic from neurogenic foot drop.
- The presence of wrist drop with foot drop should suggest MG or lead poisoning.
- The most common presentation of CMT 1A is tripping and falls due to poor clearance of toes secondary to foot drop with minimal sensory symptoms.
- Foot drop should not be confused with dystonic and spastic ankle flexion, such as in hereditary spastic paraplegia (HSP) and focal ankle dystonia. In these cases, a careful examination fails to reveal weakness of the ankle extensors, ankle reflexes are brisk, and the tone is increased in the plantar flexors.
- Copper deficiency may present with an ALS-like picture (progressive atrophy and fasciculations) plus distal sensory impairment and leucopenia. A remote gastrectomy and usage of zinc-rich denture fixative (e.g., Fixodent) are strong risk factors.
- In this case, the progressive distal asymmetrical demyelinating features with high CSF protein and monoclonal gammopathy strongly raised the possibility of DADSAM.

CASE 1.2: GAIT IMBALANCE AND APRAXIA OF EYELID OPENING

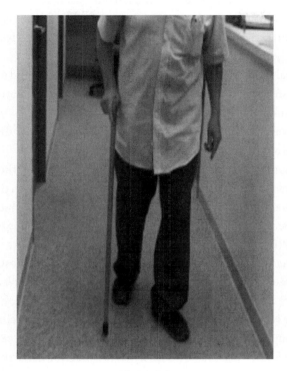

VIDEO 1.2

A 75-year-old man presented with a 4-year history of falls, which prompted his referral for neuromuscular evaluation. The symptoms were much more pronounced in the right side. Gradually he became aphasic. He had no urinary incontinence. Cognition was difficult to evaluate due to aphasia. Brain magnetic resonance imaging (MRI) revealed mild asymmetrical cortical atrophy.

This picture is typically seen in:

1. Polyneuropathy
2. Parkinson disease
3. Normal pressure hydrocephalus (NPH)
4. Corticobasal degeneration
5. Progressive supranuclear palsy (PSP)

DIAGNOSIS

- Video gait analysis: shuffling gait is characterized by markedly decreased stride length and a flat foot sliding forward during initial contact. This patient's gait also demonstrates increased lateral trunk sway and decreased reciprocal arm swing. Notice how many steps it takes to change direction 180 degrees.
- There are several areas of overlap between movement disorders and neuromuscular disorders, resulting in consultation of a neuromuscular specialist on patients with movement disorder. Examples of such an overlap:
  - Some movement disorders are associated with neuromuscular disorders such as restless leg syndrome with neuropathy.
  - Both disorders may coexist in patients by coincidence; many of these diseases are especially common in the elderly, such as neuropathy and Parkinson disease.
  - Deceptive presentations, such as dropped head syndrome, which may be confused with camptocormia or Parkinsonian posture. Sensory ataxia may be confused with gait apraxia of NPH or shuffling gait of Parkinson disease.
- Neuromuscular specialist should be aware of different manifestations and associations of movement disorders in order to detect them when referred to neuromuscular clinic.
- Gait imbalance is a common cause of a referral to neuromuscular clinic:
  - Gait is a complicated process that requires integrity of many central and peripheral mechanisms for its maintenance, such as nerves, muscles, corticospinal tracts, cerebellum, basal ganglion, cerebral cortex, and so on.
  - Normal gait also requires non-neurological elements such as skeleton, vision, vestibular apparatus, and so on.
  - Gait examination is an integral part of the examination of the nervous system; without it, the examination is never complete.
- Corticobasal degeneration in this case is suggested by the clinical and radiological asymmetry, aphasia, gait apraxia, dementia, and apraxia of the eyelid opening.
- PSP is another tautopathy that is commonly confused with this Parkinson-plus syndrome, and both can cause disorder of extraocular movements (EOMs) and gait. However, in PSP, there is predominant loss of downward gaze, mid-brain atrophy, and little, if any, asymmetry.

CASE 1.3: SENSORY ATAXIA

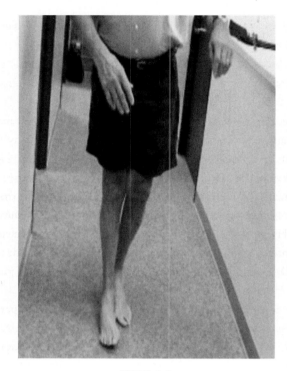

VIDEO 1.3

A 62-year-old man presented with a 1-year history of loss of balance and difficulty rising out of a deep chair. Examination is shown. In addition, he had proximal arm and leg weakness, diffuse areflexia, and no family history of significance. NCS: motor nerve conduction velocity (NCV): 30 m/sec. F-latencies: 70s. Distal motor latencies (DMLs): 8 msc. CSF protein was 150 mg/dL with increased IgG index.

Although findings of high feet arches, hammer toes, and thin legs suggested CMT, the rest of the picture is consistent with:

1. Vasculitic neuropathy (NP)
2. CIDP
3. Diabetic polyneuropathy (DPN)
4. Amyloid neuropathy
5. Alcohol-related neuropathy

DIAGNOSIS

- Painless progressive sensory ataxia with ankle dorsiflexors weakness and areflexia are very suggestive of CIDP.
- Increased IgG index in the CSF signifies increased intrathecal IgG synthesis, which in turn supports a primary inflammatory process in the peripheral or central nervous system.
- High feet arches can be congenital, and in that case they may be a marker of a congenital or hereditary neuromuscular disorder such as congenital myopathy, muscular dystrophy, CMT, and so on, or acquired due to chronic weakness of the ankle extensors, leading to unopposed action of the ankle plantar flexors. In that case, they are markers for chronic neuropathies such as CIDP. Hammer toes strongly support the former.
- CIDP may present with predominantly sensory findings such as sensory ataxia.
- CIDP is probably more common in CMT patients, and there is a suggestion that CMT may alter the antigenicity of the myelin. A similar argument is made for the inflammatory component of Duchenne muscular dystrophy (DMD) and hence a justification for steroid therapy.
- GALOP (gait disorder, autoimmunity, late onset polyneuropathy) is a variant of CIDP that is associated with IgM antibodies, mostly against sulfatide moiety, in 80% of cases, and it is usually refractory but may respond to cyclophosphamide and/or plasmapheresis.
- Sensory ataxia with preserved or brisk knee reflexes strongly argues against CIDP and suggests axonal neuropathy like vasculitis or dorsal myelopathy such as due to multiple sclerosis (MS), copper deficiency, or B_{12} deficiency.
- Ataxia is the last and least responsive of CIDP symptoms to therapy, and patients' expectations are to be lowered from the start.
- Ataxic predominantly sensory neuropathy is typically seen in Sjogren syndrome and paraneoplastic syndromes.

CASE 1.4: SPASTIC GAIT

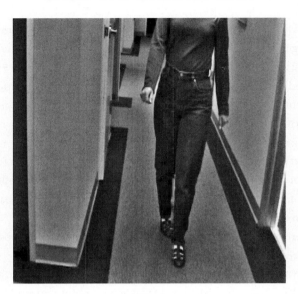

VIDEO 1.4

A 32-year-old woman presented with stiff legs, developed at the age of 15. She had no family history of significance or sensory symptoms. Gradually she developed the gait shown in the video. Her deep tendon reflexes (DTRs) were 3/4. MRI of the brain and spinal cord was normal. CSF examination was normal. Spasticity improved with Baclofen pump.

These findings are consistent with:

1. Hereditary spastic paraplegia (HSP)
2. Cerebral palsy
3. Multiple sclerosis
4. Charcot-Marie-Tooth (CMT) disease
5. Multisystem atrophy

DIAGNOSIS

- Video gait analysis: the patient's spastic gait pattern is apparent from increased adductor tone, resulting in scissoring or crossing over of the legs, as well as increased plantar flexor tone, resulting in toe walking and excessive inversion at the ankle.
- HSP is a hereditary disorder in which multiple identified genetic mutations (at least 30 mutations identified) correlate with a fairly homogeneous phenotypic syndrome characterized by spastic paraparesis.
- Patients with HSP are referred to neuromuscular clinics due to:
  - Suspicion of progressive lateral sclerosis, a variant of ALS characterized by progressive upper motor neuron (UMN) signs such as spasticity and hyperreflexia.
  - Suspicion of polyneuropathy due to gait imbalance and mild impairment of vibratory sensation in the feet.
- As in most hereditary neuromuscular disorders, the absence of a positive family history does not exclude the disorder.
- Some HSP variants, such as those caused by mutations of spastic paraplegia genes (SPG) 9, 10, 14, 15, 20, 22, 26, and 30, may display lower motor neuron (LMN) signs, further complicating differentiation from ALS.
- Slow progression, high feet arches, and mild sensory impairment in the feet due to dorsal column dysfunction favor HSP, while involvement of the arms and bulbar muscles favor primary lateral sclerosis (PLS).
- Mutation analysis can detect 60% of the autosomal dominant cases, but there is a high false negative rate. Ten percent of the sporadically affected individuals turn out to have diagnostic dominant mutations. Whole exome sequencing will hopefully increase diagnostic yield.

CASE 1.5: PAINFUL LEG SPASMS

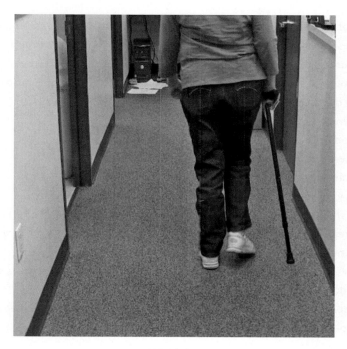

VIDEO 1.5

A 59-year-old woman presented with a 5-year history of progressive leg stiffness, painful spasms, and loss of balance. She had progressive visual failure and hearing impairment. Eye examination revealed mild optic atrophy and mild sensory impairment in the feet. She has one healthy child and several healthy sisters. No gait abnormality is reported in the parents. MRI of the brain and spinal cord, CSF examination, and electromyography (EMG) were normal. B_{12} level and copper level were normal. Very long chain fatty acids levels were normal.

The most appropriate test at this point is mutation analysis for:

1. Autosomal recessive hereditary spastic paraplegia (HSP)
2. Autosomal dominant HSP
3. ABCD gene mutations
4. Proteolpid protein gene mutations
5. SOD gene mutations

DIAGNOSIS

- The lack of affected children or siblings suggests an autosomal recessive disease.
- The optic atrophy and hearing loss suggest mitochondrial dysfunction.
- SPG 7 (paraplegin) mutations account for 4% of paraplegin mutations.
- SPG encodes a mitochondrial protein, and therefore the manifestations are protean, including optic atrophy and hearing loss.
- HSP differential diagnosis:
  - Adrenomyeloneuropathy
  - Spinocerebellar ataxia
  - Cerebral palsy
  - Primary lateral sclerosis
  - Tropical spastic paraplegia
  - Compressive myelopathies: meningeoma
- HSP is generally classified as pure or complicated.
  - In pure HSP, symptoms are generally limited to gradual weakening of the legs and impaired sensation in the feet.
  - In complicated HSP, a rare disorder, additional symptoms may include the following:
    - Peripheral neuropathy
    - Epilepsy
    - Ataxia
    - Optic neuropathy
    - Retinopathy
    - Dementia
    - Ichthyosis
    - Mental retardation
    - Deafness
    - Problems with speech, swallowing, or breathing
  - Some of these additional symptoms may be related to a separate disorder, such as diabetic neuropathy or epilepsy, rather than being directly caused by HSP.

CASE 1.6: LATERAL PELVIC TILTING

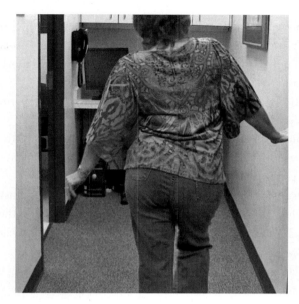

VIDEO 1.6

A 44-year-old woman presented with difficulty arising out of a chair, noticed 10 years earlier, which had gradually gotten worse. She had no sensory symptoms. A maternal cousin had a similar gait difficulty. She had no dysphagia or skin rash but had proximal weakness in the arms and legs with loss of reflexes. Creatine kinase (CK) level was 430 IU/L and EMG revealed high amplitude long duration units with a firing frequency of 25Hz in the proximal and distal muscles of the legs and arms.

This gait abnormality can be seen in:

1. Myopathies
2. Spinal muscular atrophy (SMA)
3. Congenial myasthenia gravis (MG)
4. Stiff person syndrome
5. Myelopathies

DIAGNOSIS

- Video gait analysis: pelvic drop is a sign of proximal muscle weakness (gluteus medius), which typically activates in the stance leg to hold the pelvis neutral. Exaggerated lumbar lordosis is also noted. In more advanced disease, Trendelenburg or lateral trunk movement is used to compensate for the underlying weakness.
- Lateral pelvic tilting is a postural strategy to save energy and is a feature of chronic proximal weakness, especially when it starts at an early age.
- Although traditionally it is reported as classical for muscular dystrophies, particularly DMD, it may be produced by chronic neurogenic proximal weakness such as in SMA type 3 and 4 and in congenital MG.
- It has been observed that in cases of SMA, the initial postural adjustment involves pelvic rotation, while in DMD it involves knees flexion. However, in the later stages of the disease, it may be difficult to distinguish them clinically. Even Gower maneuver may be produced by SMA.
- Spinal muscular atrophy is a group of disorders characterized by chronic and inherited degeneration of motor neurons. Unlike hereditary ALS, there are no UMN signs. Progressive muscular atrophy is a variant of ALS. It is more progressive than most SMA and it is rarely hereditary.
- SMAs are classified by age of onset and distribution of weakness; soon, classification according to molecular genetics will prevail.
  - Adult onset SMAs are:
    - Proximal SMA: 30% autosomal dominant, normal life expectancy, may have tongue fasciculations and tremors.
    - Distal SMA.
  - Kennedy disease: bulbar and proximal weakness, with sensory symptoms and elevated CK due to severe muscle cramps.
  - Scapuloperoneal SMA: asymmetric weakness of shoulder girdle and peroneal muscles leading to scapular winging and bilateral foot drop. It may be confused with FSHD.
- No treatment is available for this group of diseases.
  - A recent trial using valproic acid has failed to show a difference compared to a placebo.

REFERENCES

1. Armanda S, et al. A comparison of gait in spinal muscular atrophy, type II and Duchenne muscular dystrophy. *Gait and Posture.* 2005;21:369–378.
2. Kissel JT, et al. SMA valiant trial: a prospective, double-blind, placebo-controlled trial of valproic acid in ambulatory adults with spinal muscular atrophy. *Muscle Nerve.* 2014 Feb;49(2):187–192.

CASE 1.7: BIZARRE GAIT

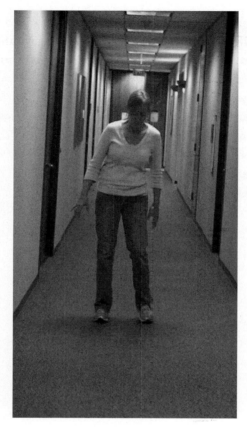

VIDEO 1.7

A 46-year-old woman presented with acute left arm and leg weakness, noticed one morning right after she woke up. Urgent brain MRI was negative. Intravenous (IV) solumedrol reversed it. Few days later she could not lift her legs; however, her examination revealed normal strength. She had normal CK level and EMG. She had no sensory or reflex changes. Her gait was demonstrated.

This gait abnormality is most likely due to:

1. Functional gait disorder (FGD)
2. Sensory ataxia
3. Cerebella ataxia
4. Myelopathy
5. Stroke

DIAGNOSIS

- FGD is common and affects mostly females.
- Gait patterns are variable and may change from one pattern to another.
- The most important clue is that the gait disorder does not conform to the description of a recognizable organic pattern and biomechanical methods of compensation.
- Falls are rare, and good strength is often demonstrated.
- Provoking factors such as stress are commonly missed, and most patients are surprised when they are told of the possible role of stress.
- Common pattern of FGDs:
  - Hemiparesis: leg dragging
  - Paraparesis: dragging of both feet
  - Ataxia
  - Dystonia
  - Myoclonus
  - Slapping
  - Robotic
  - Hesitant
  - Sudden buckling without falls
  - Waddling
  - Shaking

CASE 1.8: PROXIMAL AND DISTAL WEAKNESS

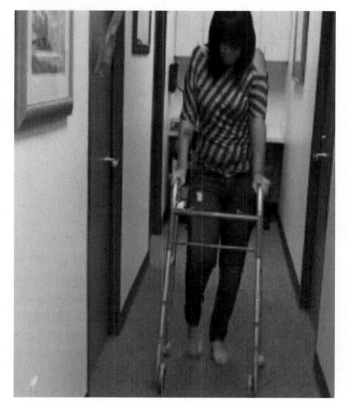

VIDEO 1.8

A 36-year-old woman presented with a 14-year history of difficulty arising out of a chair. She then had gait difficulty (shown in the video) and she progressed to a walker within 5 years. CK level was 6300 IU/L and EMG revealed evidence of irritative chronic myopathy. There was no family history. The muscle biopsy is shown in Figure 1.8.1. The biopsy also showed variation of fiber size (20–120 microns), fibers necrosis, split fibers and increased internal nuclei. She did not respond to steroids, IVIG, and methotrexate.

The following factors are consistent with dysferlinopathy:

1. Proximal and distal weakness
2. Chronic course
3. Very high CK level
4. Mild endomysial inflammation
5. No response to anti-inflammatory agents

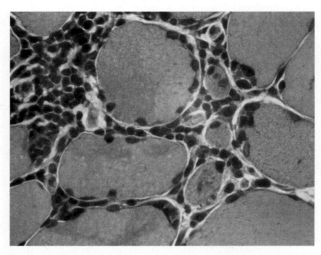

FIGURE 1.8.1 Endomysial inflammation.

DIAGNOSIS

- Waddling is a feature of chronic myopathies, more so dystrophic types. It is associated with the exaggeration of lumbar lordosis.
- Slapping due to bilateral foot drop and poor knee extension further complicates this gait.
- The chronicity and age of onset suggest a dystrophic process. More than 20 times normal CK level and dystrophic biopsy support this notion.
- Proximal and distal weakness with inflammatory and dystrophic myopathic changes is typically seen in dysferlinopathy.
- The other dystrophic myopathies that are associated with inflammatory pathology are DMD and FSHD.
- Dysferlin is an integral protein of the muscle membrane and is a target of at least 450 mutations leading to different phenotypes. It is an autosomal recessive (AR) disease.
- 6.5% of unclassified myopathies in muscle biopsies showed dysferlinopathy.
- Posterior leg muscles are affected early, leading to difficulty walking on toes. In Miyoshi variant (allelic to LGMD 2B), distal leg muscles are the main target of pathology, resulting in calves atrophy. No cardiac involvement is reported. Calves atrophy is typically seen, but hypertrophy is also reported.
- Sometimes, asymptomatic hyperCKemia is the only finding (6% of cases).
- Western-blot (WB) analysis reveals that dysferlin is reduced to 0%–20% percent in LGMD 2B and to 0 in Miyoshi myopathy.
- The disease is slowly progressive.
- Dysferlin is present in the white blood cells (WBC) and WB analysis on (WBC) is as sensitive as muscle biopsies.

CASE 1.9: LURCHING WITHOUT FALLS

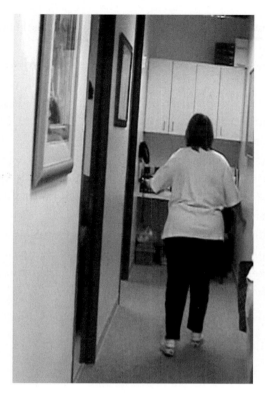

VIDEO 1.9

A 25-year-old woman who was recently divorced and had lost her job presented with the demonstrated gait abnormality. She had mild pressure like headache and chest tightness. Deep tendon reflexes were brisk but she had no weakness or sensory symptoms. At times she felt like a lump in her throat interfering with her swallowing.

This gait is likely due to:

1. Myelopathy
2. Cerebellar disorder
3. Neuropathy
4. Functional disorder
5. Trauma to the head

DIAGNOSIS

- A hysterical gait may present with monoplegia, monoparesis, hemiparesis, paraplegia, or paraparesis.
- With hysterical gait, there tends to be no leg circumduction, hyperreflexia, or Babinski sign.
- Characteristic features of a patient with hysterical gait include sudden buckling of the knees (usually without falls), swaying with the eyes closed, with a buildup of sway amplitude and improvement with distraction.
- Patients with a hysterical gait tend to drag the foot when walking rather than lift it.
- Hysterical gaits can be dramatic, with patients lurching wildly in all directions, thus demonstrating a remarkable ability to do rapid postural adjustment. In contrast, patients with true paraparesis or paraplegia tend to fall frequently.
- An unusual and illusive presentation of hysterical gait is known as astasia-abasia. In this condition, the patient is unable to turn or walk but retains normal use of the legs while lying in bed. However, atrophy of the vermis and frontal gait disorders (gait apraxia) can have similar presentation.

REFERENCE

Shaibani A, et al. Pseudoneurologic syndromes: recognition and diagnosis *Am Fam Physician*. 1998 May 15; 57(10):2485–2494.

CASE 1.10: ATAXIA AND DYSDIADOKOKINESIA

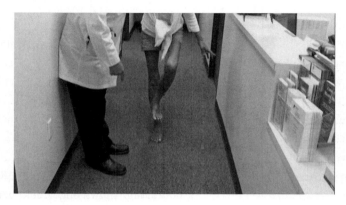

VIDEO 1.10

A 45-year-old woman presented with progressive gait imbalance for 18 months. She had also lost 30 pounds. She had no sensory, visual, or bulbar symptoms. She heavily drank alcohol 2 years earlier. She had partial pancreatectomy 3 years earlier. Examination is shown. She had normal strength, DTRs, feet sensation, and strength. MRI of the brain showed mild vermal atrophy. CSF examination was negative for oligoclonal bands (OCBs). Abdominal ultrasound (US) showed a right ovarian mass.

Which of the following antibodies is likely to be elevated?

1. Anti-Yo (anti-Purkinji cells antibodies)
2. Anti-Hu
3. Anti-Ma2
4. Anti-glutamate decarboxylase (GAD)
5. Anti-gliadin

DIAGNOSIS

- Patients with ataxia may be referred for neuromuscular evaluation.
- Cerebellar ataxia is less sensitive to loss of visual cues than sensory ataxia; therefore, Romberg sign is typically negative.
- The steps are uncoordinated and overshoot rather than hesitant and trying to find the ground.
- Other cerebellar dysfunction features are common, like nystagmus, dysmetria, dysdiadokokinesia, dysarthria, diplopia, and hyporeflexia.
- Progressive cerebellar ataxia has many causes:
  - Progressive MS: demyelianting enhancing plaques are seen in the MRI of the brain, particularity the cerebellum. CSF examination shows oligoclonal bands in 80% of cases.
  - Paraneoplastic cerebellar degeneration: this is usually subacute and is associated with weight loss and other paraneoplastic syndromes such as sensory neuropathy.
  - Hereditary SCA may exacerbate spontaneously or by stress or medications, simulating progressive picture.
  - Space-occupying lesion is to be ruled out by appropriate imaging.
  - Toxic factors such as medications and ethanol intoxication.
- Paraneoplastic cerebellar degeneration (PCD):
  - Cerebellar dysfunction due to remote effect of cancer. Molecular mimicry is the presumed mechanism.
  - PCD may precede the diagnosis of cancer by 2–5 years.
  - Ovary, uterus, breast, and lungs are the main sources. Chest X-ray and abdominal US are the most important tests in a patient with progressive cerebellar features.
  - Anti-Hu antibodies react with all neurons, but anti-Yo antibodies react only with Purkinji cells in the cerebellum.
  - Patients with anti-Yo antibodies have ovarian or breast cancers 90% of times.
  - Anti-Ri antibodies are reported in paraneoplastic encephalitis and opsoclonus in association with breast cancer and lung cancer.

CASE 1.11: GAIT DIFFICULTY WITH NORMAL EMG

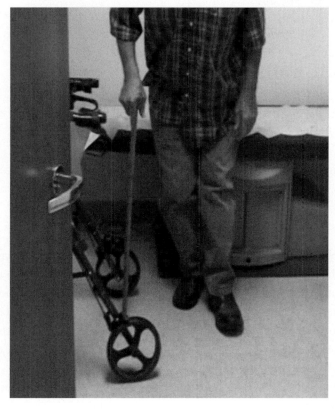

VIDEO 1.11

A 64-year-old diabetic man presented with a 2-year history of gait difficulty. He had chronic feet numbness and polyarthralgia. EMG of the proximal leg muscles was normal and CK was normal.

Which of the following tests is the most appropriate?

1. Imaging of the hips/ortho consult
2. Muscle biopsy
3. Brain MRI
4. EMG of the arms
5. Aspiration of the hip joint

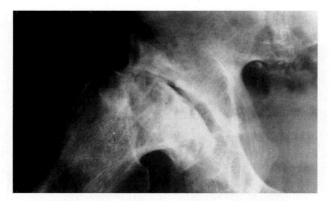

FIGURE 1.11.1 X-ray of the right hip joint revealed severe arthritis.

DIAGNOSIS

- Non-neurological disorders may be referred to neuromuscular clinics because they mimic NM disorders. Gait imbalance is the most common source of such referrals.
- This patient had a history of chronic arthritis and gradually developed restriction of hip range of motion (ROM). His examination demonstrated severe limitation of passive range of motion for hips flexion and abduction. The lack of pain (silent arthritis) was likely due to diabetic neuropathy. He also had bilateral knee arthritis, which explains his knee bending during attempted walking.
- While he had feet numbness and absent ankle reflexes suggestive of diabetic neuropathy, this gait was not neuropathic.
- His referring physician suspected myopathy. Normal CK occurs in 30% of myopathies but a normal needle examination of weak muscles strongly argues against myopathic or neurogenic weakness.
- Detailed and careful needle exploration of several weak muscles is necessary. Normal duration, amplitude, number of phases, and recruitment pattern of motor units, in multiple-tested tracks and muscles, should argue against a neuromuscular etiology. In these cases, central or non-neurological causes should be entertained.
- In chronic myopathies, motor unit estimation may be needed because compensation may lead to an apparently normal EMG picture.
- The hips X-Ray/MRI of this patient showed severe arthritis. Bilateral total hip replacement (THR) reversed his gait but maximum improvement took a year.

CASE 1.12: WIDE-BASED GAIT

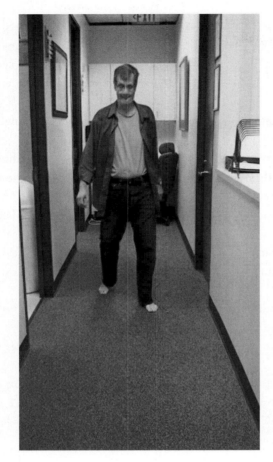

VIDEO 1.12

A 61-year-old man presented with a 10-year history of gait instability and mild feet numbness. He was a reformed alcohol drinker. In addition to what is shown in the video, examination revealed mild sensory impairment in the feet and absent ankle reflexes. There was no muscle weakness. He had a distant cousin who was wheelchair-bound due to gait imbalance. Nerve conduction study was normal.

The most likely diagnosis is:

1. Hereditary cerebellar ataxia
2. Sensorimotor neuropathy
3. Hereditary spastic paraplegia
4. Paraneoplastic cerebellar degeneration
5. Alcohol-related cerebellar atrophy

DIAGNOSIS

- Wide-based gait is a feature of vermal dysfunction, while Romberg sign signifies sensory ataxia. Therefore, this patient displays evidence of both cerebellar and sensory ataxias.
- The chronicity of the symptoms argues against paraneoplastic syndrome and suggests either alcohol-related cerebellar degeneration or hereditary cerebellar degeneration (HCD). Positive family history argues for the latter.
- Normal NCS suggests that the sensory ataxia is due to a preganglionic lesion, which is common in HCD.
- It is imperative to examine ataxic patients for other cerebellar findings such as nystagmus, dysmetria, dysarthria, and dysdiadochokinesia and to examine the dimensions of the cerebellum in the brain MRI.
- There are more than 40 types of HCD, the discussion of which is beyond the scope of this book.
- Generally, hereditary cerebellar ataxia (HCA) is classified into autosomal dominant (AD) and autosomal recessive (AR). Friedreich ataxia is the most common among the recessive ones.
- Sensory neuropathy is common in HCA types 1, 2, and 3 and in Friedreich ataxia.
- Fasciculations are characteristic of HCA type 3.
- It is important to determine the genetic type of ataxia in order to do proper genetic counseling.
- An estimated 50%–60% of the dominant hereditary ataxias can be identified with highly accurate and specific molecular genetic testing for SCA1, SCA2, SCA3, SCA6, SCA7, SCA8, SCA10, SCA12, SCA17, and DRPLA; all have trinucleotide repeat expansions in the pertinent genes.

REFERENCE

Bird TD. Gene reviews: Hereditary Ataxia Overview, February 27, 2014.

CASE 1.13: MAGNETIC GAIT

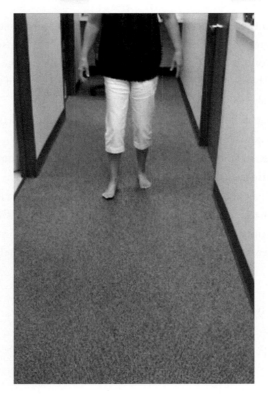

VIDEO 1.13

A 70-year-old woman presented with a 6-month history of falls and urinary incontinence. Her family noticed impaired recent memory. She had no sensory symptoms and her examination revealed normal strength and coordination. Brain MRI revealed enlarged ventricles. CSF opening pressure was 100mm/Hg. Removal of 30 ml of CSF improved gait for few days.

The gait is characterized by:

1. Waddling
2. High steppage
3. Low steppage
4. Being apractic
5. Being ataxic

DIAGNOSIS

- Gait disorders in the elderly are frequent referrals to neuromuscular clinics. Peripheral neuropathy is common in this age group, and the finding of sensory impairment in the feet is the most common cause of referral as a possible cause of the gait abnormality.
- Many in the field believe that NPH is an under-diagnosed cause of treatable dementia and frequent falls in elderly.
- The gait is characterized by difficulty making the first steps, as if the feet are glued to the ground (gait apraxia).
- There is no single reliable diagnostic test, and the same symptoms can be produced by ischemic brain disease.
- Improvement of gait and neuropsychological performance after a high-volume spinal tap is the most reliable indicator of a need for a ventriculoperitoneal shunt (VPS).
- Intrathecal injection of radionucleotide (cisternogram) to measure the appearance of the isotopes in the cerebral convexities 24–48 later has a controversial diagnostic value.

CASE 1.14: PROGRESSIVE ATAXIA

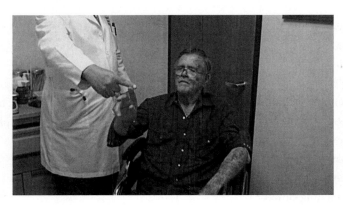

VIDEO 1.14

A 74-year-old man presented with a 6-month history of falls and slurring of speech. He had lost 15 pounds. He was a chronic smoker. He had a history of diabetic neuropathy. MRI of the brain was normal. EMG revealed moderate axonal sensorimotor neuropathy. MRI of cervical spines revealed cervical cord compression by osteophytes with intramedullary signal abnormality. Chest X-ray showed a right pulmonary nodule.

The clinical picture is highly suggestive of:

1. Diabetic polyneuropathy
2. Cervical myelopathy
3. Paraneoplastic cerebellar degeneration
4. Paraneoplastic myopathy
5. Limbic encephalopathy

DIAGNOSIS

- Patients with cerebellar ataxia may be referred to neuromuscular clinics due to suspicion of ataxic neuropathy, in particular if they have a concomitant neuropathy, usually diabetic or alcohol-related.
- Romberg sign greatly favors sensory ataxia as opposed to cerebellar ataxia because patients with proprioceptive loss rely on vision to compensate for loss of balance.
- Both cerebellar and sensory ataxias may occur simultaneously as a part of the same paraneoplastic syndrome or due to unrelated causes.
- Weight loss and history of smoking are strong risk factors for PCD.
- Cancers commonly associated with PCD:
  - Small cell lung cancer
  - Ovarian cancer
  - Breast cancer
  - Hodgkin lymphoma
- The main target of this autoimmune attack is the Purkinje cells in the cerebellum.
- Cerebellar ataxia may precede the other manifestations of cancer by up to 2 years.
- Paraneoplastic antibodies are more useful to reveal association with malignancy than to define the exact type of the malignancy, as many of them can be present in several types of paraneoplastic syndromes.
- Hu antibodies are more commonly seen in paraneoplastic sensory neuronopathy but are also reported in PCD. Small cell lung cancer is the main source.
- Reversible neuronal (Tr) antibodies are associated with lymphoma.
- Yo antibodies are associated with ovarian and breast cancers.
- Prognosis is guarded and largely depends on the underlying malignancy.

CASE 1.15: FREQUENT FALLS

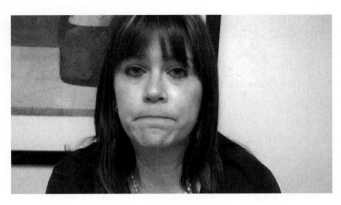

VIDEO 1.15

A lady presented with frequent falls.

These episodes are consistent with:

1. Syncope
2. Vestibular neuritis
3. Cardiac arrhythmias
4. Periodic paralysis
5. Psychogenic etiology

DIAGNOSIS

- Sudden and transient loss of muscle tone without alteration of consciousness or vertigo is called a "drop attack."
- These patients are referred to neuromuscular clinics after negative investigations for central nervous system disorders such as:
  - Brain stem ischemic
  - Hydrocephalus
  - Colloid cyst of the third ventricle
  - Atonic seizures
- The closest neuromuscular disorder to these attacks is periodic paralysis, familial or non-familial, hypokalemic or hyperkalemic.
- However, periodic familial paralysis is not that brief, and it does not happen that often without trigger factors such as exercise or high-carbohydrate diet.
- Cataplexy is usually associated with narcolepsy. Her multiple sleep latency tests were negative.
- Syncope is associated with altered consciousness.
- Dysautonomia was ruled out by a negative autonomic reflexes test.
- Cardiac arrhythmias cause blurred consciousness. Her long-term holter was negative even though she had several attacks during the recording.
- Brain stem ischemia was ruled out by brain MRI. She had no risk factors.
- Vestibular disorders were ruled out by electronystagmography (ENG) and vestibular evaluation.
- She had a history of severe anxiety attacks. Panic attacks were not likely since she denied a sense of apprehension or chest tightness or palpitation.
- The most common cause of drop attacks in the elderly is carotid sinus hypersensitivity.
- Psychogenic etiology is suspected. The problem was corrected after her anxiety was treated and the source of stress was eliminated.

CASE 1.16: CHRONIC PROGRESSIVE GAIT DISORDER WITH OPHTHALMOPLEGIA

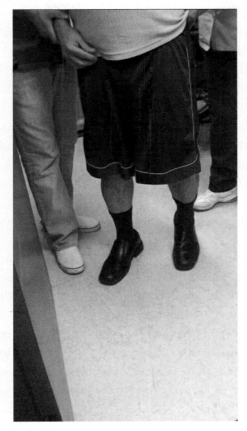

VIDEO 1.13

A 59-year-old man presented with a 3-year history of gait difficulty and frequent falls. His wife noticed clumsiness of the right arm, increased emotionality, and impairment of memory. He also developed slurring of speech. Brain MRI showed mild atrophy of the right frontoparietal lobes. Sensorimotor examination was limited by dementia and impersistence.

The most likely diagnosis is:

1. Parkinson disease
2. Progressive supranuclear palsy
3. Corticobasal degeneration (CBD)
4. Multisystem atrophy (MSA)-P
5. MSA-C

DIAGNOSIS

- Patients with ophthalmoplegia and gait instability are referred to neuromuscular clinics for suspicion of mitochondrial syndromes.
- This patient had ophthalmoplegia, severe shuffling and hesitation of gait, rigidity, hyper-reflexia, hypomimia, and dysarthria.
- The first step in evaluating ophthalmoplegia is to determine if it is central or peripheral by performing Doll's eye movement test. In this case it was central.
- The first test in evaluating neuropathy is by examining feet sensation and ankle reflexes. In this case the reflexes were brisk and the feet sensation was hard to evaluate.
- Supranuclear ophthalmoplegia is an important finding in many movement disorders. A certain degree of impairment is seen in most patients with neurodegenerative disorders with careful testing. However, it is only grossly clinically detectable in a few patients.
- PSP is notorious for causing falls due to impairment of downward gaze. In this case, gaze is impaired in all directions.
- Clinical and radiological asymmetry, dementia, and apraxia are important features of CBD, which can also cause ophthalmoplegia and Parkinsonism.
- In this case, the abnormal gait and hypomimia had suggested PD initially. However, the gait rhythm has a lower frequency than that of PD.
- Gait apraxia that is seen in NPH is a misnomer and should not be confused with leg apraxia of CBD, which is not as well studied as upper extremities apraxia. In this case, these is no leg apraxia, as the patient could not stride across a line drawn on the floor.
- Although CBD and PSP are pathologically distinct, it may be impossible to distinguish them clinically or radiologically.

REFERENCE

Hashimoto AK, et al. Analysis of gait disturbance in a patient with corticobasal degeneration. *Rinsho Shinkeigaku*. 1995 Feb;35(2):153–157.

CASE 1.17: SPASTIC GAIT

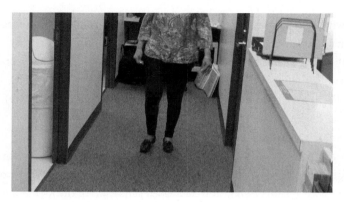

VIDEO 1.17

A 59-year-old woman presented with an 8-year history of loss of balance, falls, stiffness of the right leg, and feet numbness. She had no urinary symptoms. She had no past history of focal neurological deficit. Her symptoms progressed and she started using a cane. In addition to what is demonstrated in the video, her examination showed impaired sensation to vibration and proprioception in the feet. Cervical MRI revealed no spinal cord compression. EMG/NCS was normal.

The most appropriate next diagnostic step in this case is:

1. Brain MRI and CSF examination
2. Epidermal nerve fiber density analysis
3. Nerve biopsy
4. Autonomic reflexes testing
5. Therapeutic trial with steroids

DIAGNOSIS

- Patients with ataxia are referred for neuromuscular evaluation for neuropathy. Many of these patients turn out to have a non-neuromuscular syndrome such as:
  - Sensory ataxia due to myelopathy such as B_{12} or copper deficiency, multiple sclerosis, and so on.
  - Cerebellar ataxia such as hereditary cerebellar degeneration (HCD), paraneoplastic cerebellar degeneration.
  - Gait apraxia such as normal pressure hydrocephalus.
  - Spastic gait without sensory ataxia such as hereditary spastic paraplegia.
  - Movement disorders like Parkinson disease and Parkinson plus syndrome.
- In a patient with sensory ataxia and decreased sensation in the feet, the following should direct the attention to the spinal cord:
  - More impairment of proprioception than vibration in the feet
  - Ankle hyperreflexia
  - Positive Babinski sign: it is a good habit to check plantar responses whenever feet numbness is associated with normal or brisk ankle reflexes
  - Increased muscle tone in the legs (spastic gait)
  - Urinary urgency (although this could be due to dysautonomia)
- Skin biopsy has no practical utility in these cases. The lack of pain and the predominance of vibratory loss argue against small fibers involvement.
- This patient had multiple 3–8 mm non-enhancing periventricular white matter lesions in the brain MRI and 4 oligoclonal bands in the CSF that did not exist in the serum.
- Progressive MS can be difficult to diagnose and, unfortunately, response to the currently available preventive therapies for relapsing-remitting multiple sclerosis (RRMS) is poor in chronic progressive MS.

CASE 1.18: SENSORY ATAXIA WITH BRISK ANKLE REFLEXES

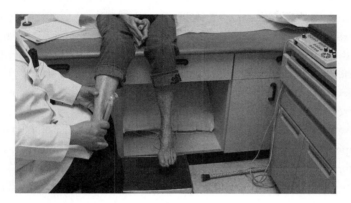

VIDEO 1.18

A 70-year-old woman presented with progressive gait instability. She had subtotal gastrectomy 10 years earlier. She used dentures. Cervical and thoracic MRIs were normal. NCS revealed mild axonal sensorimotor neuropathy. Serum B_{12} level was normal. Her peripheral WBC was 3.2 cells/mcL.

The most appropriate testing at this point is to check:

1. Copper level
2. Bone marrow aspiration
3. CSF protein
4. Selenium level
5. Zinc level

DIAGNOSIS

- Severe impairment of feet sensation to proprioception and vibration with brisk ankle and knee reflexes suggests dorsal myelopathy. Compressive causes of myelopathy were ruled out by MRIs of cervical and thoracic spines. Other causes of non-compressive dorsal myelopathies were ruled out, including B_{12} deficiency. NCS also showed axonal sensorimotor neuropathy. We are dealing with a case of myeloneuropathy.
- Small fiber neuropathy is usually associated with feet pain instead of sensory ataxia, normal reflexes, and normal NCS.
- There have been an increasing number of myeloneuropathy cases reported in association with copper deficiency.
- Risk factors:
  - Remote gastrectomy: copper is absorbed in the stomach and proximal jejunum.
  - Usage of high zinc–content fixative for dentures. The high zinc content competes with copper and drives its level down.
  - Poor nutritional status
- Leucopenia is common in copper deficiency and it is an important diagnostic clue in neurological cases.
- Copper deficiency may also present with muscle atrophy and fasciculations similar to ALS.
- The myeloneuropathy may improve with oral or IV copper replacement, but residual deficit is common. Hematological abnormalities are more amenable to correction.
- The exact role of copper in neural growth and regeneration is not clear.
- It is important that copper level is checked, along with B_{12} level, in all cases of myeloneuropathies.
- All patients with gastrectomy should be supplemented with micronutrients and vitamins consistently starting right after surgery.

CASE 1.19: FAMILIAL GAIT SPASTICITY

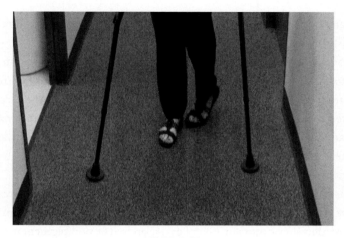

VIDEO 1.19

A 72-year-old woman presented with a 10-year history of slowly progressive gait imbalance. EMG revealed mild sensory neuropathy. She had two brothers with similar symptoms. B_{12} and copper levels were normal. Testing for HSP autosomal dominant and recessive mutations were negative. MRI of the cervical and spinal cord was normal.

The following tests are appropriate except:

1. Serum very long-chain fatty acids (VLCFA) level
2. Examination of the affected brothers
3. ATP-binding cassette, sub-family D (ALD), member 1 (ABCD1) gene mutation
4. Serum fasting cortisol level
5. Serum zinc level

DIAGNOSIS

- Video demonstrated and examination showed spastic gait, hyperreflexia, positive Babinski signs, sand sensory ataxia.
- VLCFA level was very high and pathogenic ABCD1 mutation was found.
- X-linked adrenomyeloneuropathy is an important but rare cause of chronic progressive myeloneuropathy in adults, and heterozygous cases that affect women are even rarer.
- It is caused by mutation of ABCD1 gene. It codes for adrenoleukodystrophy protein, which is an important component of the peroxisomal membrane and allows for the passage of very long-chain fatty acid to the perioxisomes.
- More than 650 mutations are found in this gene.
- Symptoms start in the second to fourth decades with spastic paraparesis and sensory ataxia and hyperreflexia. Associated axonal neuropathy and dysautonomia are common. Adrenal insufficiency occurs in 70% of cases, leading to skin pigmentation, hypotension, gastrointestinal (GI) upset, and generalized weakness. Cortisone level is low.
- Female carries display symptoms at age 20–55 years as late onset myelopathy. Adrenal insufficiency is rare despite low corticosteroids reserve.
- Steroid replacement is effective for adrenal insufficiency but there is no cure for myelopathy.
- All non-compressive myelopathies should be tested for VLCFA level and if high, for ABCD1 mutations, especially if there is a family history of affected males and features of adrenal insufficiency.
- Although it is an X-linked disease, women may be affected later in life and are usually misdiagnosed as multiple sclerosis or familial spastic paraparesis.
- This disease is allelic with adrenal leukodystrophy that affects children.

CASE 1.20: ATAXIA AND NIGHT BLINDNESS

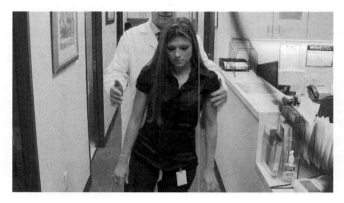

VIDEO 1.20

A 32-year-old woman presented with visual impairment since childhood; she was diagnosed with retinitis pigmentosa. A few years later, she developed loss of balance and feet numbness; she was diagnosed with neuropathy. She continued to get worse. MRI of the brain and spinal cord was negative. She had a sister with similar symptoms and a brother who was diagnosed with CMT. Retinal exam is shown (Figure 1.20.1). EMG revealed mild sensory neuropathy.

Mutation of which of the following genes may explain this picture?

1. MT-ATP6 gene
2. FLVCR1 gene
3. PHYH gene
4. TTPA gene
5. SCA-2 gene

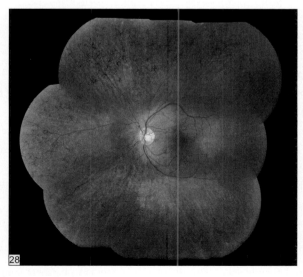

FIGURE 1.20.1 Fundoscopic examination.

TABLE 1.20.1 Genetic conditions associated with ataxia, neuropathy, and retinitis pigmentosa

Disease	Chromosome	Gene	Inheritance
• NARP (neuropathy ataxia, and retinitis pigmentosa)	• mtDNA	• *MT-ATP6*	• Maternal
• PHARC (polyneuropathy, hearing loss, ataxia, retinitis pigmentosa, and cataract)	• 20p11.21	• *ABHD12*	• AR
• Ataxia with isolated vitamin E deficiency	• 8q12.3	• *TTPA*	• AR
• Refsum disease	• 10p13	• *PHYH*	• AR
• Abetalipoproteinemia	• 4q23	• *MTP*	• AR
• CDG1A (congenital disorder of glycosylation type IA)	• 16p13.2	• PMM2	• AR
• Spinocerebellar ataxia 2*	• 12q24.12	• SCA2	• AD
• PCARP (posterior column ataxia, with retinitis pigmentosa)	• 1q32.2	• FLVCR1	• AR

DIAGNOSIS

- Video demonstrated and examination showed severe impairment of proprioception and vibration sensation in the feet and mild loss of pinprick (PP) sensation, absent ankle and knee jerks, and sensory ataxia. Fundoscopic examination revealed retinitis pigmentosa (Figure 1.20.1).
- The above listed possibilities have to be considered in patients with ataxia, neuropathy, and retinitis pigmentosa (Table 1.20.1).
- Nerve conduction study revealed sensory neuropathy.
- In this case most of the possibilities were ruled out:
  - Genetic testing for neuropathy, ataxia, and retinitis pigmentosa (NARP) was negative.
  - Phytanic acid level was normal.
  - The patients did not have cerebellar ataxia or hearing loss.
  - Transferrin glycosylation pattern was normal.
  - Serum lactate and pyruvate levels were normal.
  - Mitochondrial genome was entirely normal.
  - Vitamin E and abetalipoprotin B levels were normal.
- Sequencing of feline leukemia virus subgroup C cellular receptor (FLVCR1) revealed two pathogenic mutations.
- PCARP is an AR disorder characterized by ataxia, neuropathy, and retinitis pigmentosa. Mutation of FLVCR1 gene is reported at least in four families to cause this syndrome. The gene is mapped to 1q32.
- FLVCR1 is a heme exporter. Its role in causing neurological damage is not clear.

REFERENCE

Ishiura H, et al. Posterior column ataxia with retinitis pigmentosa in a Japanese family with a novel mutation in FLVCR1. *Neurogenetics* 2011;12:117–121.

CASE 1.21: NEUROPATHY AND NYSTAGMUS

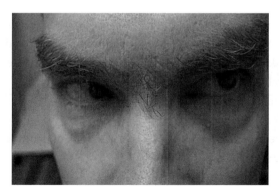

VIDEO 1.21

A 50-year-old man presented with gait imbalance since age 20. As he grew up, he had to turn his head to different directions to see, despite preservation of EOM. Neuro-ophthalmological consult concluded that he had oculomotor apraxia (OMA). Progressively he relied on a wheelchair for mobility. Brain MRI showed cerebellar atrophy. He also had numbness of the feet, and the NCS revealed axonal sensorimotor neuropathy. CK level was 780 IU/L and alpha-fetoprotein was elevated in the blood.

These findings are typically seen in:

1. Freidrieck ataxia
2. Ataxia with oculomotor apraxia
3. Spinocerebellar ataxia-1
4. Machado Joseph disease
5. Spinocerebellar ataxia and sensory neuropathy

DIAGNOSIS

- The video demonstrated bilateral ptosis and severe fixed ophthalmoplegia and proximal weakness.
- Congenital myasthenic syndromes (CMS) are due to genetic mutations in genes that encode for proteins at the neuromuscular junction.
- They may be classified as presynaptic, synaptic, and postsynaptic.
- The most common CMS include:
  - Presynaptic CMS: choline acetyl transferase deficiency. It often causes a severe phenotype with episodes of apnea.
  - Synaptic CMS: acetylcholinesterase deficiency. It results in over-activation of the neuromuscular junctions as well as autonomic ganglia. Thus the pupils are often non-reactive in these patients. Electrodiagnostic testing may show a repetitive CMAP.
  - Postsynaptic CMS: acetylcholine receptor (AChR) subunit mutations (including alpha, beta, delta, and epsilon), muscle-specific kinase (MuSK), rapsyn, and Dok-7. Mutation of AChR subunits may result in three different physiological effects:
    - AChR deficiency: fatal or severe
    - Early AChR closure (fast channel)
    - Prolonged AChR opening (slow channel)
- Epsilon mutation is not fatal because expression of the fetal gamma-AChR subunit will partially rescue the phenotype.
- Fast channel is a milder defect that would result in partially attenuated receptor response to acetylcholine. The phenotype may be improved with acetylcholinesterase inhibitors (e.g., pyridostigmine) and 3,4 diaminopyridine.
- Patients with slow channel syndrome demonstrate a repetitive CMAP on electrodiagnostic testing. Due to prolonged opening of these channels, agents that partially block the AChR, such as quinine, quinidine, or fluoxetine, often provide symptomatic improvement.
- Mutations in Dok-7 and Rapsyn have been demonstrated to exhibit a later onset limb-girdle distribution weakness.

CASE 2.3: DELAYED EYES OPENING

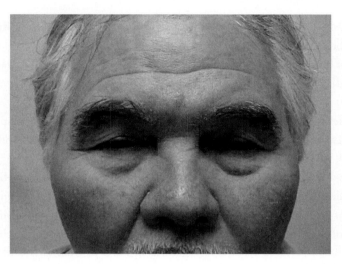

VIDEO 2.3

A 60-year-old man presented with a 4-year history of falls. In addition to what was shown in the video, he had a normal Doll's eye movement and cerebellar ataxia.

The most likely diagnosis is:

1. Parkinson disease
2. Multisystem atrophy-P
3. Progressive supranuclear palsy (PSP)
4. Chronic progressive external ophthalmoplegia (CPEO)
5. Multisystem atrophy–C

DIAGNOSIS

- Examination revealed supranuclear ophthalmoplegia, eyelid apraxia, hypomimia, and mild cerebellar ataxia.
- Apraxia of lid opening (ALO) is a nonparalytic motor abnormality characterized by difficulty initiating the act of lid elevation after lid closure despite preservation of muscle strength.
- These patients are referred to neuromuscular clinics because they are suspected of having ptosis and along with ophthalmoplegia, myasthenia gravis and mitochondrial disease are suspected.
- Delayed eye opening after voluntary closure is not a feature of ptosis. Relief of apraxia by sensory cues such as touching the face is characteristic. This phenomenon of *geste antagoniste* might be useful in distinguishing apraxia of lid opening from myotonia of eyelids.
- The lack of forceful closure differentiates ALO from blepharospasm. However, 10% of blepharospasm patients may display features of ALO as well. This explains the lack of response to botulinum toxin in some cases of blepharospasm.
- ALO is a feature of many neurodegenerative disorders such as Parkinson disease, Huntington disease, corticobasal degeneration, and progressive supranuclear palsy.
- Doll's eye movement was preserved in this case, indicative of supranuclear nature.
- Axial rigidity and frequent falls are suggestive of PSP. Impairment of downward gaze may have been present early in the course and was replaced by a total ophthalmoplegia as the disease progressed.
- Like PSP, corticobasal degeneration is a tauopathy, but it is usually associated with features of cortical dysfunction such as aphasia, dementia, and alien hand syndrome.

CASE 2.4: PTOSIS IN THE ELDERLY

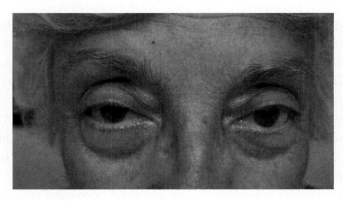

VIDEO 2.4

A 70-year-old woman presented with a long-standing, non-fluctuating bilateral ptosis without diplopia.

The most likely diagnosis is:

1. Hyperthyroidism
2. Ocular MG
3. Dermatochalasis
4. Oculopharyngeal muscular dystrophy
5. Levator dehiscence

DIAGNOSIS

- Elderly with droopy eyelids are often referred to neuromuscular clinics, especially when their chronic ptosis starts blocking their vision. It is common that patients do not think much about chronic ptosis and consider it to be normal. The appearance of other age-related symptoms such as declined vision, dryness of eyes, and decreased swallowing due to dryness are prompting factors for evaluation.

- The most accurate measurement of ptosis is marginal reflex distance (MRD), which is the distance between the lower eyelid margin and the center of pupillary light reflex with the eye in the primary gaze. MRD of more than 2 mm or an asymmetry of more than 2 mm indicates ptosis.

- Ptosis is a common presentation to both emergency rooms and neurology clinics, and it has a wide variety of causes, ranging from serious ones like posterior communicating artery aneurysm to benign ones like dehiscence of the LPS.

- The upper eyelid normally covers 20% of the cornea. The position of the eyelid is affected by gaze (droops slightly with lateral gaze, elevated with upward gaze, and droops with downward gaze) and by the state of arousal (elevated with full arousal and droops with drowsiness).

- Levator dehiscence is the most common cause of lowered eyelids and occurs mostly in the elderly.
  - The eye crease is created by insertion of the LPS to the pretarsal plate and is normally less than 5 mm.
  - When the LPS tendon is disinserted from the tarsal plate, the eyelid droops and becomes thin but maintains normal range of motion.
  - Such a disinsertion of the LPS may be caused by trauma to the eye such as eye surgery (cataract extraction) or non-surgical trauma as simple as eye rubbing.
  - Hard contact lenses can also cause it. In these cases the ptosis appears acutely, leading to an alarm in the family, but most of the time, a history of chronic drooping is present.
  - High skin crease (more than 7 mm) is a characteristic feature. Typically the eyelid has a normal range of motion.
  - Failure to diagnose this condition may lead to unnecessary investigations. Correction is simple by surgical shortening of the LPS or insertion of tendon sling. Ptosis props are rarely useful.

CASE 2.5: UNIDIRECTIONAL DIPLOPIA

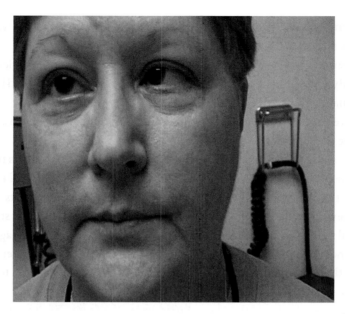

VIDEO 2.5

A 48-year-old woman presented with acute horizontal right gaze diplopia with no ptosis or diurnal variation.

Which muscle is weak as detected by the demonstrated test?

1. Right medial rectus (MR)
2. Right lateral rectus (LR)
3. Left MR
4. Right LR
5. Right superior oblique (SO)

DIAGNOSIS

- Blepharospasm may be a source of referral to neuromuscular clinics due to confusion with ptosis. Confusion of ptosis with blepharospasm can be dangerous; ptosis may be due to MG where botulinum toxin is contraindicated.
- Blepharospasm is a forceful involuntary eye closure due to focal dystonia of orbicularis oculi. It is usually bilateral but can be asymmetric.
- In 20% of cases it starts unilaterally.
- It should be differentiated from ALO, which is due to failure of LPS to contract. Both may coexist.
- Blepharospasm increases under bright light and during time of stress; hence it may interfere with driving.
- Ptosis may do the same under these conditions. About two-thirds of patients are rendered functionally blind by blepharospasm.
- Blepharospasm may be associated with mandibular and facial dystonia (Meige syndrome).
- The spasms may be transiently alleviated by pulling on the upper eyelid or the eyebrow, pinching the neck, talking, humming, yawning, singing, sleeping, relaxing, reading, concentrating, looking down, and performing other maneuvers or sensory tricks (*geste antagonistique*).
- The cause of blepharospasm may be impairment of the mechanism of blinking. Normally blinking is reduced by 74% during reading and increased 100% during conversation. Normal individuals blink more frequently during conversation than during rest. In blepharospasm, the pattern is reversed.

REFERENCE

Gomez-Wong E, Marti MJ, Tolosa E, Valls-Sole J. Sensory modulation of the blink reflex in patients with blepharospasm. *Arch Neurol.* 1998;55:1233–1237.

CASE 2.7: SYMPTOMS RESOLVED AFTER PRAYER

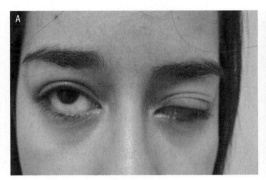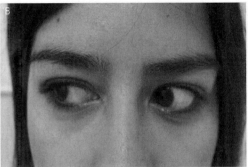

VIDEO 2.7

A 18-year-old woman presented with intermittent left ptosis and fatigable diplopia (video 2.7A) with positive binding AChR antibodies. She refused treatment and her symptoms resolved with prayer (video 2.7B), only to come back 6 months later.

The following is true about resolution of symptoms with prayer:

1. It is due to spontaneous resolution of MG.
2. It is against the diagnosis of MG.
3. MG symptoms are often induced by prayer.
4. It occurs only in seropositive cases.
5. Prayer should be tried first and then medication.

DIAGNOSIS

- MG, like other autoimmune diseases, may spontaneously remit temporarily or permanently.
- The natural history of MG was studied in a cohort of 73 patients before the era of disease-modifying agents.
- 22% of patients went into a complete clinical remission, 18% had improved considerably, 16% had improved moderately, 16% had not changed, 3% had deteriorated, and 29% had died, including 8 who had thymoma.
- Another study found a remission rate of 10% and a death rate of 35% in 360 patients. Over half of the deaths occurred in the first 3 years. Twenty percent improved and 30% had not changed and 5% got worse.
- Spontaneous remission is more likely as time passes, and complications are more likely during the first 3 years of the diagnosis.
- Remission rate without treatment is 5%, 24%, 33%, and 41% at 1, 3, 5, and 10 years.
- There are no clear factors that are associated with more chances of spontaneous remission.

REFERENCES

Beghi E, et al. Prognosis of MG: a multicenter follow up study of 844 patients. *Journal of Neurological Sciences*. 1991;106:213–220.

Oosterhuis HJGH. The natural course of myasthenia gravis: a long term follow up study. *Journal of Neurology, Neurosurgery, and Psychiatry*. 1989;52:1121–1127.

CASE 2.8: MYASTHENIA WITH DILATED PUPIL

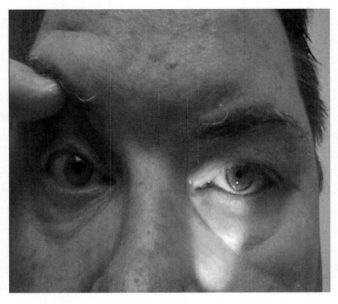

VIDEO 2.8

A 56-year-old man presented with fluctuating right ptosis, which started after a recent cataract surgery. He had diplopia due to left medial rectus weakness that started after a right orbital trauma that mandated a major reconstructive surgery several years earlier, but the diplopia had worsened recently. The ptosis was temporarily relieved with an ice pack, and the diplopia resolved when the ptosis was complete. The right pupil was not reactive to light. AChR Ab titer was positive.

Which of the following argues against the diagnosis of MG?

1. The response of ptosis to ice pack
2. The resolution of diplopia when the ptosis is complete
3. The appearance of ptosis after surgery
4. The pupillary abnormality
5. None of the above

DIAGNOSIS

- Patients who are referred for neuromuscular evaluation for suspected MG may end up having different diagnoses.
- About 10% of cases referred by neuro-ophthalmologists to the Nerve and Muscle Center of Texas for confirmation of MG turned out to have an alternative diagnosis, and the misdiagnosis was enhanced by negative brain magnetic resonance imaging (MRI).
- On the other hand, even in serologically proven MG, one may discover irreconcilable findings such as dilated pupil(s). Patients may not be aware of these findings, or they do not give a relevant history because they do not think it is important.
- This patient had fixed and dilated right pupil from an old trauma that required orbital surgery, which also changed the anatomy of the orbital muscles. However, the right ptosis is a new finding that prompted a search for MG.
- Resolution of diplopia with complete ptosis is expected, as vision from one eye is not enough to produce diplopia. Monocular diplopia is more likely an image split due to retinal, corneal, or lenticular disease rather than actual diplopia. Very rarely, a central lesion produces monocular diplopia. The double image does not appear when viewing thorough a pinhole.
- The appearance of symptoms of MG after physical or emotional trauma is not unusual. This is the case with all autoimmune diseases.

CASE 2.9: APRAXIA OR PTOSIS?

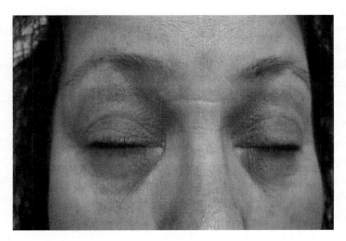

VIDEO 2.9

A 41-year-old woman presented with a 3-month history of diplopia and difficulty opening her eyes. Her examination reveals multidirectional diplopia and weakness of the orbicularis oculi. She also had difficulty opening her eyes once voluntarily closed, suggesting eyelid apraxia. Myasthenia gravis serology was positive and she responded to steroids.

Apraxia of lid opening (ALO):

1. Can be seen with blepharospasm
2. Can be seen in isolation
3. Can be confused with eyelid myotonia
4. Can be confused with ptosis
5. Never responds to botulinum toxin

DIAGNOSIS

- Upper eyelid ptosis (drooping) is an important manifestation of MG. It is diagnosed when the upper eyelid covers more than 20% of the cornea.
- ALO is the inability to open the eyes with preservation of strength and understanding of the command.
- Ptosis may be confused with ALO, but there is usually weakness and fatigability of the levator palpebral superioris (LPS) and orbicularis oculi (OO).
- ALO is due to abnormality of supranuclear control of eyelid elevation, which requires the activation of the LPS and concurrent inhibition of the OO activity.
- Botulinum toxin injections to the pretarsal muscle may be useful when there is an associated blepharospasm, and it may benefit ALO due to pretarsal motor activity persistence but not when ALO is due to involuntary LPS inhibition.
- It is crucial that ALO is not confused with ptosis from MG because botulinum toxin is contraindicated in the latter.

CASE 2.10: MYASTHENIC SYMPTOMS WORSENED WITH STEROIDS

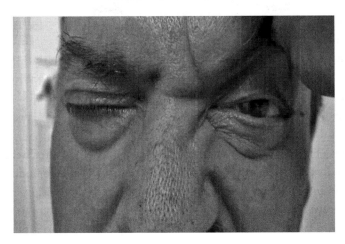

VIDEO 2.10

A 55-year-old man presented with a 6-month history of evening diplopia and dysarthria. Examination is shown. Resting forced vital capacity (FVC) was 50% of normal.

The most specific test for this condition is:

1. AChR Ab titer
2. Repetitive nerve stimulation test
3. Computed tomography (CT) scan of the chest
4. Single-fiber electromyography (SFEMG)
5. Brain MRI

In MG, when respiratory function is compromised, initiation of high-dose steroids:

1. May precipitate respiratory failure
2. Usually improves bulbar symptoms within 24 hours
3. Does not worsen dysphagia
4. Reduces the need for monitoring respiratory functions

DIAGNOSIS

- Worsening of myasthenic symptoms occurs in 25%–50% of cases, and it is severe in 7% of cases. Patients with bulbar dysfunction should be closely monitored after initiation of steroids. If bulbar function is remarkably compromised, initiation of steroids is safer under observation in the hospital or is preceded by IVIG or plasmapheresis.

- The cause of such worsening is not clear. Steroids are known to worsen certain neuromuscular conditions and therefore they are contraindicated in Guillain-Barré syndrome and multifocal motor neuropathy with conduction block.

- Elevation of the eyebrows in the ptotic side is a normal compensatory mechanism. Depression of the eyebrow would suggest a functional (psychogenic) etiology.

- Ptosis in myasthenia can happen without diplopia or bulbar dysfunction. Diagnosis can be difficult to make, especially given that serology and RNS are negative in 40% of cases. Tensilon test can be helpful in these cases. SFEMG on the weak levator palpebral superioris or orbicularis oculus is more helpful (if negative) to rule out the disease. A positive test is not specific.

- Fluctuation is an important sign in MG, but in chronic cases, muscles may become fixed by fibrosis. A therapeutic steroid trial may be needed to settle the diagnosis.

- The risk of thymoma is the same; therefore, computed tomography (CT) scan of the chest should be ordered, even in MG cases that present with ptosis only.

CASE 2.15: WATCH OUT FOR STEROIDS COMPLICATIONS

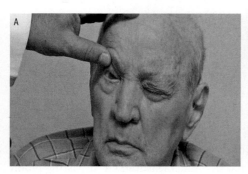 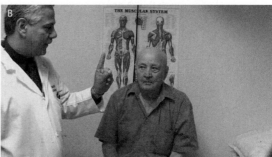

VIDEO 2.15

A 92-year-old man presented with a 2-month history of subacute bilateral ptosis and diplopia. AChR Ab titer was elevated (video 2.15A). CT scan of the chest was negative. He did not respond to pyridostigmine, but 4 weeks after oral prednisone 60 mg a day, his symptoms resolved. He was able to walk, swallow, chew, and see without problems (video 2.15B). He rarely needed pyridostigmine.

The most appropriate next step in management of this case is:

1. Add a steroid sparing agent such as azathioprine.
2. Change pyridostigmine to 120 mg five times a day.
3. Continue the same dose of prednisone for a year.
4. Start tapering prednisone to the lowest most effective maintenance dose.
5. Thymectomy.

The prednisone was tapered to 15 mg every other day. A year and a half later, he fell and fractured a femur, which was complicated by deep venous thrombosis (DVT).

Long-term complications of steroids include all of the following except:

1. Cataract
2. Osteoporosis
3. Proximal weakness
4. Hypertension
5. Neuropathy

DIAGNOSIS

- While high-dose oral prednisone is effective in 90% of cases of MG, complications are common, and close monitoring is required, especially in the elderly.
- 25% of patients develop complications, which are dose and duration dependent:
  - Osteoporosis: the most serious long-term complication. Menopausal smoking women are at the highest risk. The risk of femoral fracture after a minor fall is high, and the outcome can be devastating. Weight-bearing exercises such as walking are to be encouraged. A diet rich in calcium, protein, and vitamin D is recommended. An annual bone density scan and supplementation with calcium, 1000 mg a day, Vitamin D3 1000 units a day, and etidronate 5 mg a day are recommended.
  - Diabetes mellitus (DM): dietary control and periodic measurement of fasting blood sugar (FBS) or hemoglobin A1c (HbA1c) are advised.
  - Easy bruisability and muscle weakness
  - Glaucoma and cataract
  - Gastric erosion and indigestion
  - Fluid retention
  - Mood changes, depression, insomnia
  - Weight gain
  - Infection including thrush
  - Hypertension
  - Hypertrichosis
  - Acne
- Monitoring of body weight, blood pressure, serum glucose, skin integrity, muscle strength, dietary measures, yearly bone density scan, treatment of insomnia and anxiety, avoidance of mixing with sick children, and so on, are useful preventive measures.
- Very often patients ask if they can take influenza vaccination. Influenza vaccination is not contraindicated in MG. Immunosupression or recent treatment with plasmapheresis or intravenous gammaglobulin may reduce the effectiveness of vaccinations.

CHAPTER 3

DIPLOPIA

CASE 3.1: WEAK LATERAL RECTUS

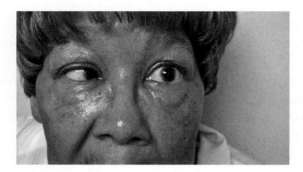

VIDEO 3.1

A 72-year-old African-American woman presented with fluctuating diplopia to lateral gaze bilaterally and elevated acetylcholine receptors antibody titer. She had incidental left Bell palsy 2 years earlier.

Bilateral weakness of the lateral rectus muscle is a feature of:

1. Amyotrophic lateral sclerosis
2. Myasthenia gravis (MG)
3. Benign intracranial hypertension
4. 1 and 2
5. 2 and 3

DIAGNOSIS

- The video shows bilateral weakness of lateral rectus.
- About 50% of cases of myasthenia gravis present with ocular symptoms such as ptosis and diplopia.
- 75% of these cases will generalize. Generalization mostly occurs in the first 2 years after the diagnosis and only rarely occurs later.
- Most patients with generalized myasthenia gravis have ocular involvement.
- The cause for preferential involvement of EOM is not clear.
  - EOM are smaller, contract faster than extremity muscles, and have fewer muscle fibers per motor neuron. Such a delicate and fast contraction ability predisposes them to fatigue.
  - It has been proposed that the types of antibodies that attack EOM are different from the ones that affect extremity muscles.
  - The function of EOM is delicate, and even minor weakness can cause symptoms due to misalignment of the EOM that leads to diplopia.
- EOM involvement in MG is so variable that several diseases can be mimicked and the diagnosis thus may be delayed, especially when the weakness is limited to the EOMs.
- The EOM involvement is usually bilateral but asymmetrical.
- The most common patterns are:
  - Weakness of the superior oblique and inferior rectus (65%). This leads to vertical diplopia that occurs with sustained upward gaze.
  - Single EOM involvement occurs in 12% of cases.
  - Superior oblique weakness causes diagnostic confusion with 4th cranial nerve palsy.
  - Lateral rectus weakness may mimic 6th cranial nerve palsy.
  - Medial rectus weakness mimics 3rd cranial nerve palsy.
  - Inferior rectus weakness.
  - Bilateral medial rectus involvement can mimic internuclear ophthalmoplegia.
  - Rarely, bilateral lateral rectus weakness may happen, leading to diagnostic confusion with chronic intracranial hypertension such as seen in benign intracranial hypertension.
  - Benign intracranial hypertension does not cause ptosis.
  - Third cranial nerve palsy causes complete ptosis, but the weakness in this case affected only the lateral rectus and none of the muscles innervated by the 3rd cranial nerve.
  - Diplopia is not a feature of amyotrophic lateral sclerosis (ALS).

CASE 3.2: MEDIAL RECTUS WEAKNESS

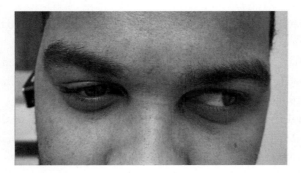

VIDEO 3.2

A 25-year-old man presented with ocular myasthenia gravis controlled with oral steroids. When the steroids were discontinued, he developed weakness of the medial recti without ptosis.

Isolated weakness of the medial recti can be caused by:

1. Myasthenia gravis (MG)
2. Bilateral 3rd cranial nerve palsy
3. Multiple sclerosis
4. Clivus meningeoma
5. Benign intracranial hypertension

DIAGNOSIS

- The medical recti are susceptible to fatigue in myasthenia gravis and they can be the presenting feature of the disease.
- Lateral gaze may reveal weakness of the medial rectus of the adducted eye and nystagmus of the abducted eye that gets coarser with more fatigue of the ipsilateral lateral rectus. This is called pseudo internuclear ophthalmoplegia.
- Sustained lateral gaze for 30–45 seconds is usually enough to produce weakness of MR in MG.
- Holding visual target too close to the patient may produce failure of convergence, which may not be an abnormal sign.
- Moving the visual target away would resolve the produced diplopia if it was due to convergence failure; it would worsen if it was due to MG.
- Associated weakness of the orbicularis oculi strongly favors myasthenia as a cause of MR weakness.
- In most instances, ptosis, fatigable dysarthria, dysphagia, and weakness of mastication muscles make it easy to diagnose MG, but difficulties arise when the weakness is limited to EOM muscles and when fluctuation is not prominent and abnormal serology is absent.
- Single-fiber electromyography (SFEMG) is useful, especially if a weak facial muscle (frontalis, orbicularis oculi) is tested. Testing EOM themselves with SFEMG is not an option in clinical practice.
- Clivus meningeoma and benign intracranial hypertension do not cause bilateral medial rectus weakness.

CASE 3.3: POSITIVE EDROPHONIUM TEST

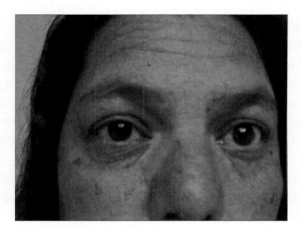

VIDEO 3.3

A 63-year-old woman presented with fatigable painless binocular diplopia on left lateral gaze only with reported right ptosis with partial response to edrophonium and negative MG serology. Initial brain magnetic resonance imaging (MRI) was normal. Three months later she developed nystagmus, and a repeat brain MRI was abnormal (Figure 3.3.1).

Edrophonium test:

1. Is 90% specific for MG
2. If negative, excludes MG
3. Is always negative in brain stem glioma
4. Can be positive in pseudoptosis

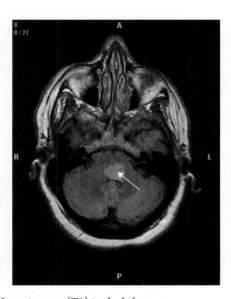

FIGURE 3.3.1 Brain MRI: Hyperintense (T1) in the left pons.

DIAGNOSIS

- This patient was found to have a brain stem glioma.
- Edrophonium inhibits acetylcholinesterase and thus prolongs the availability of acetyl-choline at the neuromuscular junction, which in turn results in enhanced muscle strength.
- Onset of action is within 30 seconds and duration of action is up to 5 minutes.
- 2 mg of edrophonium is injected intravenously and if there is no unwanted reaction such as bradycardia, the remaining 8 mg is injected.
- Facial muscle twitching, lacrimation, salivation, sweating, and flushing are indicators of action.
- Pyridostigmine should be stopped for 24 hours before the procedure.
- Atropine should always be available to reverse severe muscarinic side effects. It will not affect nicotinic side effects.
- A placebo arm is advocated, but its impact on the outcome of the test is questionable.
- It is imperative that a measurable weak muscle is monitored for action such as ptosis or weak EOM.
- A nonspecific response such as improvement of fatigue is not essentially a positive response.
- It is 70% sensitive and very nonspecific. False positive response can happen in ALS, brain tumors, and pseudoptosis.
- In the last 10 years, the performance of this test has dramatically declined in most neuro-muscular practices due to its poor contribution to the diagnosis of equivocal cases and the availability of SFEMG.

CASE 3.4: MYASTHENIA MIMICKER

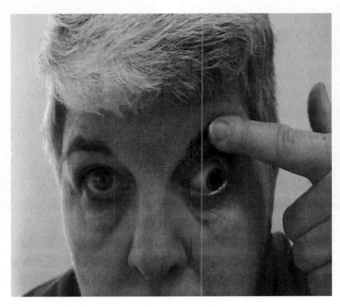

VIDEO 3.4

A 65-year-old woman presented with progressive left ptosis and medial rectus weakness. She had negative MG serology, brain MRI, and magnetic resonance angiogram (MRA) of the brain. She responded partially to pyridostigmine. Three months later she developed headache and left mydriasis. A repeat brain MRI and MRA showed a left cavernous sinus lesion.

Cerebral arteriogram revealed carotid cavernous sinus fistula (Figure 3.4.1 and Figure 3.4.2). She improved after embolization.

The following findings are not typical for MG:

1. Severe headache
2. Frontal numbness
3. Nystagmus
4. Morning diplopia
5. All of the above

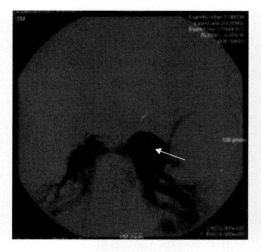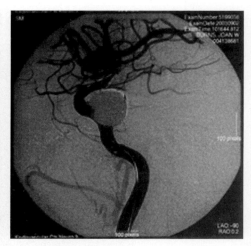

FIGURE 3.4.1 AND FIGURE 3.4.2 Left carotid cavernous fistula (CCF) before (3.4.1) and after (3.4.2) embolization.

DIAGNOSIS

- CCF is formed by abnormal communication between the carotid artery and the cavern-ous sinus. It is more common in young age groups and is mostly traumatic.
- If the cavernous sinus connects to the intracavernous carotid artery, the flow in the fistula would be high. If the cavernous sinus connects to branches of the carotid system within the adjacent dura, the flow would be low (cavernous dural fistula). This is more common in elderly women and is usually spontaneous and idiopathic. Genetic connective tissue disease and hypertension are risk factors. The cavernous sinus contains cranial nerves 3, 4, 5, and 6. Only V1 and V2 of the trigeminal nerve pass through the cavernous sinus. These nerves are affected in the following fashion:
  - Diplopia is the presenting feature in 85% of cases
  - Cranial nerve 6 is involved in 50%–85% of cases
  - Cranial nerve 3 is involved in 67% of cases
  - Cranial nerve 4 is involved in 49% of cases
- Headache occurs in 53%–75% of cases and retro-orbital pain occurs in 35% of cases; this argues against myasthenia gravis, which is usually painless. Mild frontal pain may occur in MG due to compensatory activity of frontalis.
- Proptosis and facial sensory symptoms are common
- Loss of vision occurs in 33% of cases due to orbital venous congestion and vitreous bleeding.
- After successful closure, cranial nerve dysfunction usually improves over months and persists in a minority.
- While atypical, morning diplopia and nystagmus of a weak medial rectus muscle can be seen in MG.

REFERENCE

Kim MS, Han DH, Kwon OK, Oh CW, Han MH. Clinical characteristics of dural arteriovenous fistula. *J Clin Neurosci.* 2002;9(2):147.

CASE 3.5: UNIFYING DIAGNOSIS IS NOT ALWAYS POSSIBLE

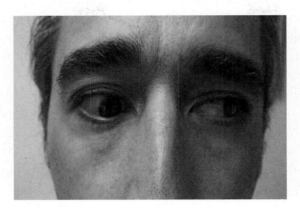

VIDEO 3.5

A 44-year-old man presented with a 6-year history of partially steroid responsive proximal weakness, recurrent steroid responsive oligoarthritis, painless fatigable vertical diplopia, and dysphagia. Creatine kinase (CK) was 450 IU/L and muscle biopsy revealed endomysial inflammation. Rheumatoid factor was positive. Brain MRI is shown (Figure 3.5.1).

Facioscapulohumeral muscular dystrophy (FSHD) is suggested by the examination and confirmed by mutation analysis, but it does not explain:

1. Diplopia
2. Pectoralis atrophy
3. Oligopolyarthritis
4. Inflammation in muscle biopsy
5. Horizontal clavicles

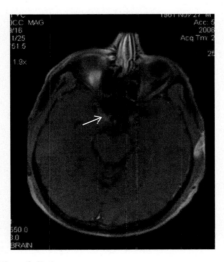

FIGURE 3.5.1 Brain MRI with gadolinium.

DIAGNOSIS

- While the primary diagnostic strategy in neurology is to find a unifying diagnosis to multiple findings, it is sometimes difficult to find one explanation or disease process for all clinical and laboratory data. In such situations, the neuromuscular specialist should be aware of atypical presentations and of exclusive findings of certain diseases.
- This patient has three disorders:
  1. FSHD: pectoralis atrophy, deltoid hypertrophy, horizontal clavicles, and proximal weakness suggested this. The diagnosis is genetically confirmed. Diplopia is not expected as FSHD does not involve EOMs. Endomysial inflammation is typically seen in these patients.
  2. Rheumatoid arthritis: this is suggested by consistently steroid responsive oligoarthritis and very high rheumatoid factors. Endomysial inflammation is also seen in some cases.
  3. Apical cavernous meningioma: diplopia and dysphagia raised the possibility of MG. Initial brain MRI was negative, but the repeat MRI a few months later was abnormal. It showed asymmetry and possible mass in the right cavernous sinus c/w meningioma. Meningioma may compress the 3rd, 4th, or 6th cranial nerves, depending upon its location and size. Retro-oribital pain, ocular redness, and proptosis are seen if the tumor attains certain size. Meningeoma was confirmed and treated with radiation.

CASE 3.6: PENALTY FOR CORRECTION OF WRINKLES

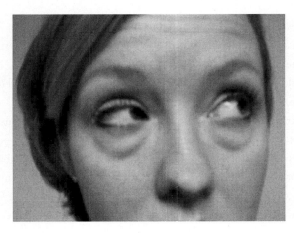

VIDEO 3.6

A 32-year-old female presented with blurring of vision 3 days after receiving botulinum toxin (BT) injections in the face for cosmetic reasons.

BT mechanism of action:

1. Blocks the postsynaptic acetylcholine receptors (AChR)
2. Blocks acetylcholine esterase in the neuromuscular junction
3. Inhibits the release of acetylcholine from the presynaptic terminal
4. Inhibits sodium channels on muscle membrane
5. 1 and 3

DIAGNOSIS

- The video showed bilateral ptosis and multidirectional diplopia.
- Cosmetic botulinum toxin (BT) injection has become the most common application of BT in medicine over the last decade.
- BT is also used to treat focal dystonia (e.g., blepharospasm, cervical dystonia, spasmodic dysphonia), hemifacial spasm, spasticity, and migraine.
- BT inhibits acetylcholine release from presynaptic nerve terminals and therefore prevents the contraction of the related muscles.
- Complications of BT can be functionally and cosmetically significant.
- Diplopia and ptosis are more common the closer the injection is to the eyes. Low frontalis injections may cause ptosis due to involvement of the levator muscle. The toxin affects the surrounding muscles by diffusion, and it does not have to be injected into them to cause weakness.
- Doses of different BT preparations are not interchangeable, and the use of the wrong conversion factor may lead to overdose.
- Side effects, like good effects, appear within a week and last for 2–3 months. It is important to explain the temporary nature of these potential side effects to the patients.
- Most patients who are referred to neuromuscular centers do not volunteer information about cosmetic use of BT because they are not aware of a relationship between their symptoms and these injections, or they are embarrassed or afraid they will be thought vain.
- Patients with neuromuscular transmission disorders should be warned against any form of BT and should be told about the possibility of precipitating additional weakness or myasthenic crisis.
- Neuromuscular complications of BT are due to weakness of the affected muscles and may include:
  - Diplopia and ptosis from periorbital injections
  - Facial weakness from injection of facial muscles for hemifacial spasm or for cosmetic reasons
  - Dysphagia from cervical injections, mostly for dystonia
  - Jaw ptosis from injections of the masseter and pterygoid and sometimes lower facial muscles
  - Weakness of finger flexors and extensors from injections for tremors and focal dystonia
  - Foot drop from injections for spasticity and focal foot dystonia

CASE 3.7: OBLIQUE DIPLOPIA

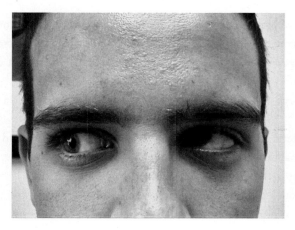

VIDEO 3.7

A 17-year-old-man presented with a 1-year history of non-fatigable oblique diplopia. Examination is shown. MG serology and brain MRI were normal.

These findings are typical of:

1. Abducent palsy (6th cranial nerve)
2. MG
3. Oculomotor palsy (3rd cranial nerve)
4. Trochlear palsy (4th cranial nerve)
5. Convergence spasm

DIAGNOSIS

- Trochlear nerve palsy (TNP) may result from lesions anywhere along the course of the nerve from its nucleus in the midbrain to the superior oblique (SO) muscle.
- It has the longest intracranial course and is the only nerve with a dorsal exit from the brainstem.
- It passes through the cavernous sinus and enters the SO muscle via the superior orbital fissure.
- The primary action of the SO is intorsion (to move the eye down and in) of the globe and the secondary action to depress the globe maximally on medial gaze.
- Vertical diplopia that resolves with head tilt to the other side is typical, and patients assume a chronic head tilt to avoid diplopia. Looking downward, such as when going downstairs, may lead to falls due to diplopia.
- On examination, the affected eye is tilted upward (ipsilateral hypertropia), with extorsion. The deviation is greater with the maximum action of the affected muscle (left SO weakness appears with right gaze) and when the head is tilted ipsilaterally.
- Clinical diagnosis of unilateral 4th cranial nerve palsy is done by three steps:
  1. Determination of the hypertrophic eye: if the left eye is hypertrophic, the weakness may be in the left SO, or IR, or right SR, or IO.
  2. Production of diplopia: if diplopia occurs with right gaze in a left hypermetropic eye, the weakness is then either left SO or IR.
  3. Head tilt: if diplopia worsens with head deviation to the same side of the hypertrophic eye, then the weakness is in that side SO.
- Causes: congenital (40%), traumatic (30%), and idiopathic (30%). The long intracranial course of the nerve carries a long risk for involvement by tumors and increased intracranial pressure (ICP).
- Important causes of 4th cranial nerve palsy seen in neuromuscular clinics:
  - Cavernous sinus pathology: other nerves are usually affected: 3rd, 5th, 6th
  - Retro-orbital pathology: there is usually proptosis and conjunctival congestion
- Important neuromuscular differential diagnoses of 4th cranial nerve palsy:
  - MG: SO weakness can be the only manifestation of MG. Usually other EOMs are affected at some point, especially MR. Weakness of facial muscles and ptosis are common. Fluctuation of diplopia is an important clue.
  - Thyroid ophthalmopathy

CASE 3.8: OPHTHALMOPLEGIA WITH ELEVATED CK

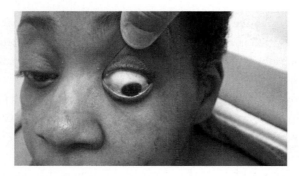

VIDEO 3.8

A 41-year-old woman presented with a 4-week history of diplopia, ptosis, dysphagia, dysarthria, dyspnea, chewing fatigability, skin rash, proximal weakness, and weight loss. Chest X-ray revealed ground glass appearance, and the CPK level was 1560 U/L. EMG revealed paraspinal and proximal fibrillations and myopathic units. Muscle biopsy revealed inflammatory myopathy. AChR antibodies titer was elevated. CT chest showed no mediastinal abnormalities. She remitted with prednisone and azathioprine.

MG with elevated creatine kinase (CK) to more than 10 times normal occurs in:

1. Giant cell myositis
2. Musk MG
3. Brachio-cervical inflammatory myopathy
4. Paraneoplastic syndrome
5. 1 and 3

DIAGNOSIS

- Mild elevation of creatine kinase (less than 500) occurs in 10% of MG patients.
- More severe elevation is not common and should raise the possibility of an associated myopathy, especially if there is severe proximal weakness and myopathic EMG (both can happen in MG, but not typically).
- The most important two neuromuscular syndromes that cause high CK and MG are:
  1. Giant cell myositis (granulomatous myopathy, thymoma, and MG)
  2. Brachiocervical inflammatory myopathy (BCIM)
- BCIM:
  - Inflammatory myopathy that affects proximal arm more than leg muscles and is associated with ptosis and ophthalmoplegia in 30% of cases and increased AChR Ab in 30% of cases.
  - Weakness of posterior neck muscles, dysphagia, respiratory failure, myalgia, skin rash, and weight loss are characteristic features.
  - Associated mixed connective tissue disease, Sjogren syndrome, rheumatoid arthritis (RA), and scleroderma are common.
  - Irritative myopathy is seen in EMG, and CK may be up to 15x normal.
  - Muscle pathology shows evidence of primary inflammatory myopathy. Perivascular and perimysial mononuclear infiltration, MAC deposition, and B cells predominance, along with skin rash and interstitial lung disease, suggest similar disease to dermatomyositis (DM).
  - The more severe involvement of bulbar, cervical, and upper extremities more than lower extremities and the associated ptosis and ophthalmoplegia are not typical for DM and warrant recognition of a different entity. However, the associated MG can explain all these findings. These could be two autoimmune disorders affecting the same patient.
  - Steroid therapy is usually effective.

REFERENCE

Pestronk A, Kos K, Lopate G, Al-Lozi MT. Brachio-cervical inflammatory myopathies: clinical, immune, and myopathologic features. *Arthritis Rheum.* 2006 May;54(5):1687–1696.

CASE 3.9: WHICH EOM IS FIRST AFFECTED IN MYASTHENIA GRAVIS?

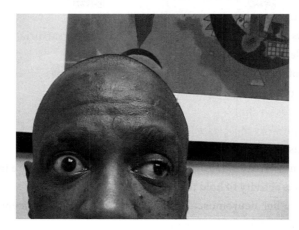

VIDEO 3.9

A 43-year-old man presented with subacute diplopia and ptosis that developed over a few weeks. Examination revealed more involvement of the medial than lateral recti and triceps than biceps muscles.

In MG, the following patterns of muscle fatigability are commonly seen:

1. Neck extensors more than flexors
2. Medial recti more than lateral recti
3. Triceps more than biceps
4. Ankle extensors more than ankle flexors
5. All of the above

DIAGNOSIS

- Thyroid eye disease is one of the most common differential diagnosis of ocular myasthenia gravis.
- Lid lag due to hyperactive levator palpebral superioris (LPS) from hyperthyroidism may give a false impression of exophthalmos.
- Unlike MG, thyroid ophthalmopathy (TO) is associated with lid lag instead of ptosis most of the time. However, when exophthalmos is severe and once hyperthyroidism is treated and lid lag improves, ptosis may develop due to levator dehiscence from protrusion pressure. Ptosis in these cases is non-fluctuating and the crease line is elevated.
- Infiltration of orbital tissue and EOM with inflammatory cells is the pathological hallmark of TO. The primary antigen is TSH receptors, against which antibodies are formed and can be measured commercially.
- TO is the presenting feature of Graves disease in 20% of cases, and appears during the disease in 40% of cases and after the disease is diagnosed in 20%. TO may occur in Hashimoto thyroiditis and is sometimes isolated.
- TO and MG may coexist, leading to more orbital complications and diagnostic delay.
- Enlargement of EOM is the radiological hallmark of TO. CT or MRI scan of the orbits can easily demonstrate this.
- TO may worsen after treatment of Graves disease, and it may threaten vision.
- Steroids treatment usually helps. Local radiotherapy and decompressive surgery may be needed in refractory cases to save vision.
- Retro-orbital masses and EOM myositis are important differentials for TO in addition to MG.

CASE 3.11: DIPLOPIA AND RETRO-ORBITAL PAIN

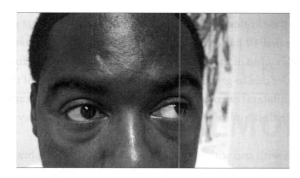

VIDEO 3.11

A 33-year-old man presented with a 2-month history of acute right retro-orbital pain and photophobia that was followed by binocular multidirectional diplopia and right forehead numbness.

The most appropriate test is:

1. Repetitive nerve stimulation test
2. MRI of the brain and orbits
3. AChR antibody level
4. CT scan of the chest
5. Lumbar puncture

CHAPTER 4

OPHTHALMOPLEGIA

CASE 4.1: DIPLOPIA AND BRISK REFLEXES

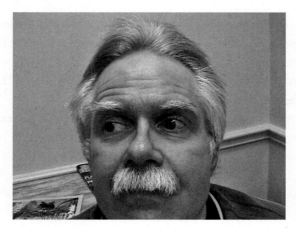

VIDEO 4.1

A 40 year-old-man presented with recurrent episodes of transverse myelitis and optic neuritis who gradually developed diplopia to lateral gaze bilaterally, which was not fatigable. Deep tendon reflexes (DTRs) including jaw jerk were brisk.

The following is (are) correct regarding the video findings:

1. Internuclear ophthalmoplegia (INO)
2. The side of the INO is named after the abducted eye.
3. Bilateral lesion of medial longitudinal fasciculus (MLF)
4. Pathognomonic of multiple sclerosis (MS)
5. A complication of treatment of MS

DIAGNOSIS

- INO is one of the most localizing signs in neurology. It is due to a lesion of MLF, which connects the nuclei of the 6th and 3rd cranial nerves and is located in the dorsal part of the pons and midbrain.
- The most common cause of INO is cerebrovascular disease, followed by MS. Other causes include tumors, infections, and trauma.
- INO presents with horizontal diplopia, and examination reveals weakness of the ipsilateral adducted eye and nystagmus of the contralateral abducted eye.
- The cause of nystagmus is not clear. It may be an adaptive response to weakness of the adducted eye.
- Myasthenia may mimic INO. Medial rectus weakness is common in myasthenia gravis (MG), and adaptive response of the fatigable contralateral lateral rectus (LR) sometimes induces abnormal movement that mimics nystagmus.
  - In the presence of other manifestations of MS and MG, diagnosis is not difficult.
  - However, when these symptoms occur in isolation, the most important differentiating sign is sparing of convergence response in INO due to the preserved integrity of the convergence center.
  - In peripheral medial rectus (MR) weakness, however (3rd cranial nerve palsy, MG, etc.), such a response is affected.
- INO is named after the side of the adducted eye (medial rectus).

CASE 4.2: FLOPPY BABY WITH OPHTHALMOPLEGIA

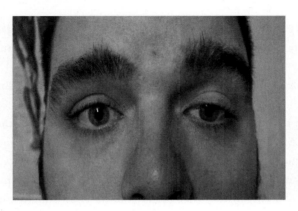

VIDEO 4.2

A 27 year-old-man who was born as a floppy baby presented with ophthalmoplegia. Gradually, he was able to walk, but proximal weakness, ophthalmoplegia, and ptosis continued. Repetitive spinal accessory nerve stimulation (RNS) produced a decremental response of the ipsilateral trapezius. He responded to pyridostigmine well.

The following deficits are reported in post-synaptic congenital myasthenic syndrome (CMS):

1. Choline acetyltransferase deficiency
2. Dok-7 mutation
3. Acetylcholine esterase deficiency
4. Epsilon mutation
5. Sodium channelopathy

DIAGNOSIS

- CMS is a rare group of disorders that can be confused with seronegative MG, especially when encountered in adult population. They do not respond to immunomodulation or suppression.
- Fatigable weakness of ocular, bulbar, and limb muscles is present since infancy or early childhood.
- Some may improve but exacerbate by infection, medications, and other sources of stress.
- All types of CMS decrement with 2–3 Hz stimulation, but presynaptic forms increment with high frequency stimulation.
- Some muscles may be spared; therefore, testing multiple muscles is important.
- The presence of family history is helpful, but its absence is not exclusive. Most of these syndromes are autosomal recessive.
- Postsynaptic CMS is the most common type, and the most common of this type is primary deficiency of AChR or primary kinetic defect of these receptors. Rapsyn, epsilon, and Dok-7 mutations are the next most common.
- Quinidine is contraindicated in all CMS except slow channel syndrome.
- Pyridostigmine is helpful in most cases but should be avoided in endplate acetylcholinesterase deficiency, where ephedrine and albuterol are usually beneficial.
- 3,4-DAP is useful in most cases except slow channel syndrome.
- In an adults with fatigable weakness, the following findings would support CMS:
  1. Onset of symptoms at or shortly after birth
  2. Decremental electromyogram (EMG) response to 3 Hz stimulation
  3. Negative double MG serology
  4. Lack of clinical improvement with immunosuppression
  5. Presence of family history of the same

CASE 4.3: BULGY EYES AND HEAT INTOLERANCE

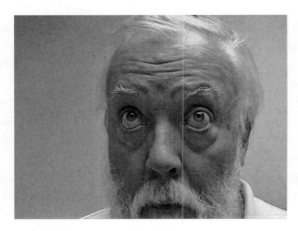

VIDEO 4.3

A 60-year-old-man presented with progressive weight loss, diplopia, and heat intolerance. His examination is shown.

Thyroid ophthalmopathy causes diplopia by:

1. Fatty infiltration of the retro-orbital tissue
2. Slowing neuromuscular transmission
3. Enlargement of the extraocular muscles (EOMs)
4. Paralyzing oculomotor nerves
5. Cavernous sinus pathology

DIAGNOSIS

- Examination showed mild restriction of eye movements, exophthalmos, swelling of the eyelids, and congestion of conjunctiva.
- Diplopia and ophthalmoparesis that are produced by thyroid ophthalmopathy (TO) are often confused with MG.
- The volume of extraocular muscles and retro-orbital tissue is increased due to accumulation of glycosaminoglycans, mostly hyaluronic acid. This leads to accumulation of fluid and bulging of the eyes, thus interfering with the function of the EOMs and venous drainage of the orbits.
- EOM are enlarged and distorted by inflammatory infiltration and edema. Auto-antibodies to different parts of retro-orbital tissue, including EOM, are detected in the serum of these patients.
- The activation of T-cells is mostly initiated by thyroid-stimulating hormone (TSH) receptor antigen. This notion is supported by the recovery of TSH receptors mRNA in the orbital tissue.
- There is a correlation between the severity of the ophthalmopathy and the serum level of TSH receptor antibodies.
- TO is more common in women, but it tends to be more aggressive in men.
- Family history, presence of other autoimmune diseases, and smoking are risk factors for TO.

CASE 4.4: HOW LONG SHOULD MG BE TREATED?

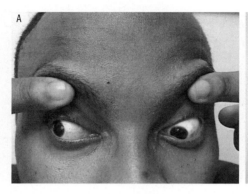 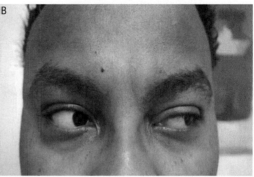

VIDEO 4.4

A 35 year-old-man presented with fatigable horizontal diplopia that improved with rest. AChR antibody titer was elevated. He responded to pyridostigmine for a year, then he had to increase the dose to 540 mg a day with minimal benefit. He refused steroids. After a year he could not drive anymore due to complete ptosis at night. Three months after steroid therapy, the ophthalmoplegia and ptosis resolved (video 4.4B).

Evidence from clinical trials supports a safe discontinuation of prednisone after a remission for:

1. Two years
2. Four years
3. One year
4. Five years
5. No evidence

DIAGNOSIS

- The video showed ophthalmoplegia and severe bilateral ptosis.
- There are no guidelines or evidence-based medicine regarding the duration of treatment of MG.
- Most experts try to wean off medications after 2 years of remission.
- 25% of patients may remain in remission after discontinuation of immunosuppression after 2 years.
- Thymectomy may increase this percentage by 35%, but more specific information will be available from the currently active thymectomy trial in 2016.

CASE 4.5: OPHTHALMOPLEGIA AND RESPIRATORY FAILURE

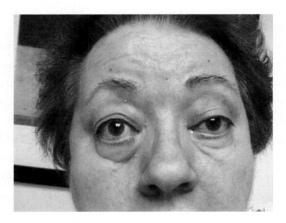

VIDEO 4.5

A 61-year-old-woman presented with blurring of vision and leg weakness that had started 2 years earlier. AChR and MuSK antibody testing was negative. Repetitive nerve stimulation showed no significant decrement. A diagnosis of seronegative generalized MG was considered, and she was treated with corticosteroids and thymectomy. Only subjective response to therapy was noted. One year later she developed respiratory failure and she was found to have the demonstrated abnormalities. Serum lactate and pyruvate levels were five times greater than normal, and left biceps muscle biopsy was abnormal (Figure 4.5.1 and Figure 4.5.2). Mutation analysis on muscle tissue revealed several pathogenic mitochondrial mutations. She died from respiratory failure.

Which of the following features are more consistent with chronic progressive external ophthalmoplegia (CPEO) than with MG?

1. Subacute onset
2. Increased levels of serum lactate and pyruvate
3. Response to steroids
4. Ragged red fibers in muscle biopsy
5. Age of patient

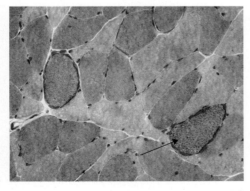

FIGURE 4.5.1 Modified Gomori trichrome stain (100X).

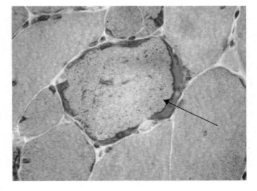

FIGURE 4.5.2 Modified Gomori trichrome stain (400X).

DIAGNOSIS

- The muscle biopsy pictures demonstrated ragged red fibers.
- Although this patient was initially thought to have MG, she ultimately was diagnosed with CPEO. Both MG and mitochondrial disease may present with ophthalmoplegia and ptosis. CPEO is associated with myopathy; however, mild myopathic features may also sometimes be seen on needle EMG of patients with myasthenia. Patient with mitochondrial disease may report periodic worsening and subjective improvement with steroids. These features can make distinction between the two disorders challenging.
- Although diffuse chronic weakness of EOM does not typically cause diplopia, periodic worsening triggered by external or internal factors may lead to diplopia.
- CPEO may be confused with MG, congenital myasthenic syndrome, oculopharyngeal muscular dystrophy (OPMD), and progressive supranuclear palsy. The presence of multisystemic manifestations such as deafness, seizures, strokes, cardiac conduction defects, retinal pigmentary changes, and neuropathy should favor the diagnosis of mitochondrial disorders.
- Chronic progressive external ophthalmoplegia usually presents with ophthalmoplegia and ptosis, with or without proximal weakness.
  - Onset usually occurs in the 4th decade but can be at any age.
- KSS is similar to CPEO, but the onset is usually before age 20 years and there are cardiac conduction defects and retinal pigmentary changes. It is more progressive.
- CPEO is a heterogeneous group of disorders: it can be sporadic, maternally inherited (deletion of large mitochondrial gene) which constitutes 50% of cases, or autosomal dominant or recessive (nuclear mutations).
- Mild creatine kinase (CK) elevation is common but is not required for the diagnosis. EMG is either normal or shows mild myopathic changes.
- Serum resting lactate and pyruvate are increased in 60% of cases.
- Cerebrospinal fluid (CSF) lactate and pyruvate are more sensitive but not specific, as they can be increased in strokes and seizures.
- Muscle tissue is still ideal for the diagnosis of mitochondrial mutations due to segregation of mutated mitochondria in muscle. However, if nuclear mitochondrial mutations are suspected (autosomal POLG mutations, MNGIE, etc.), peripheral blood may be as good as muscle tissue.
- Muscle biopsy usually shows ragged red fibers, the pathological hallmark of mitochondrial disorders.

CASE 4.6: DEMYELINATING NEUROPATHY WITH OPHTHALMOPLEGIA

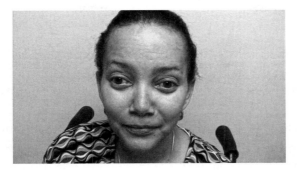

VIDEO 4.6

A 25 year-old-woman presented with progressive generalized weakness and loss of balance. She was found to have ophthalmoplegia, ataxia, and areflexia. CSF protein was slightly increased, and motor nerve conduction velocities were moderately decreased. She was diagnosed with Miller Fisher syndrome. Past medical history was remarkable for chronic abdominal distension and childhood seizures. Also, as a child, she became deaf after being treated with neomycin for a urinary tract infection. Brain MRI is shown (Figure 4.6.1).

Muscle biopsy is expected to show:

1. Myopathic changes
2. Polyglucosan bodies
3. Ragged red fibers
4. Red-rimmed vacuoles
5. Cytoplasmic inclusion bodies

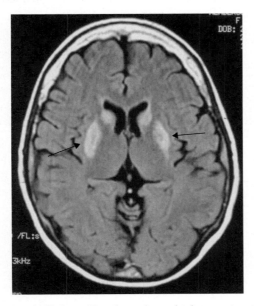

FIGURE 4.6.1 Brain MRI: revealed bilateral basal ganglionic high-intensity signals.

DIAGNOSIS

- The video shows ophthalmoplegia, deafness, areflexia, and proximal weakness. This, along with seizures, neuropathy, and MRI findings, raised the possibility of mitochondrial disorder.
- Mitochondrial diseases have a high predilection for organs with high metabolic rate such as muscle, brain, and nerves.
- Although peripheral neuropathy occurs in more than 50% of cases, it is rarely the presenting symptom.
- Most of the time, the polyneuropathy is axonal, but a demyelinating variant similar to Charcot-Marie-Tooth (CMT) disease and chronic inflammatory demyelinating neuropathy is reported.
- MNGIE syndrome has an associated polyneuropathy in 30% of cases; however, less than 5% are demyelinating.
- In this case, the subacute deterioration, areflexia, and moderate asymmetrical demyelinating neuropathy with ophthalmoplegia and ataxia led to an erroneous diagnosis of Miller Fisher syndrome.
- Deafness and seizures suggested mitochondrial disease. Gastrointestinal (GI) disturbances with demyelinating neuropathy raised the possibility of MINGIE.
- Subacute deterioration of mitochondrial disorders may be induced by medication, infection, or stress.
- Plasma thymidine phosphorylase elevation is important but not required for the diagnosis of MINGIE.
- Cases of mitochondrial disease erroneously diagnosed as CMT disease are reported. Hereditary neuropathies with negative genetic testing and history of hearing impairment or seizures should be considered for mitochondrial disorders, especially MINGIE, neuropathy, ataxia, and retinitis pigmentosa (NARP), and POLG1 and RRM2B mutations.
- Muscle biopsy revealed myopathic changes and many ragged red fibers.
- This case had MINGIE caused by RRM2B mutation.

REFERENCE

Shaibani A, MD, et al. Mitochondrial neurogastrointestinal encephalopathy due to mutations in RRM2B. *Arch Neuro.* 2009 Aug;66(8):1028–1032.

CASE 4.7: OPHTHALMOPLEGIA AND HEART BLOCK

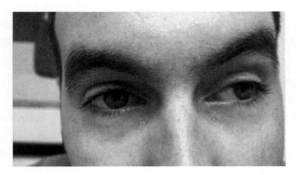

VIDEO 4.7

A 29-year-old-man presented with a 3-year history of blurring of vision. There was no visual decline, dysphagia, dyspnea, or leg weakness. There was no family history. Retinal exam was normal and electrocardiogram (ECG) revealed second-degree heart block. MG serology was negative.

The most likely diagnosis is:

1. Myasthenia gravis (MG)
2. Chronic progressive external ophthalmoplegia
3. Oculopharyngeal muscular dystrophy
4. Congenital myasthenic syndrome
5. Progressive supranuclear palsy

The most likely findings will be:

1. Hyperphosphorylated tau protein accumulation
2. Multiple small mitochondrial deletions
3. Epsilon mutation
4. A single large mitochondrial deletion
5. Nuclear inclusions

DIAGNOSIS

- Video showed partial ophthalmoplegia and ptosis with normal facial strength.
- Onset of KSS typically occurs before age 20 years, and death may occur in the 4th decade.
- KSS is a multisystemic disease with variable tissue involvement due to heteroplasmy.
- The following clinical features may be present:
  - Progressive external ophthalmoplegia and ptosis
  - Pigmentary degeneration of retina: visual loss is mild and occurs in 50% of cases
  - Heart block: usually occurs years after the development of ophthalmoplegia and leads to syncope and even sudden death
  - Dysphagia (50%)
  - Mitochondrial myopathy (90%)
  - Sensorimotor neuropathy (10%)
  - Deafness (95%)
  - Ataxia (cerebellar or sensory) (90%)
  - Encephalopathy (seizures, strokes, dementia)
  - Endocrinopathy: impaired glucose tolerance, hypothyroidism, hypoparathyroidism.
- Laboratory and imaging findings:
  - Lactic acidosis due to anaerobic metabolism
  - Mild CK elevation, myopathic EMG
  - Brain MRI: white matter changes in the basal ganglia and thalamus.
  - Ragged red fibers in muscle pathology in 98% of cases. MtDNA mutation is detected in muscle.
  - High CSF protein
- Genetics: 80% of cases are due to a single large MtDNA mutation. Most cases are sporadic.
- Treatment: There is no cure. Monitoring of ECG and early pacemaker placement, screening for and treatment of diabetes mellitus (DM), hypothyroidism, and oculoplasty are examples of medical interventions that are needed in some of these patients.

CASE 4.8: PTOSIS AND ANISOCORIA

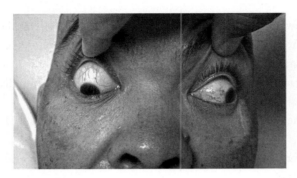

VIDEO 4.8

A 63-year-old-man presented with droopy eyelids and diplopia. Examination is shown. AChR antibody titer was remarkably high.

Pupillary abnormalities in patients with MG could be due to all of the following except:

1. Physiologic anisocoria
2. Myasthenia gravis (MG) itself
3. Prior ocular trauma
4. An independent optic neuropathy
5. Tonic pupil

DIAGNOSIS

- The video showed weakness of medial rectus bilaterally, moderate left ptosis, and anisocoria. The right pupil is slightly larger and less reactive than the left one.
- Unlike presynaptic neuromuscular disorders such as botulism and Lambert Eaton syndrome, dysautonomia is not a feature of MG. Therefore, pupillary changes are not expected and should strongly argue against the diagnosis of MG.
- However, some patients have unrelated pupillary abnormalities that may cloud the diagnosis of MG.
  - The most common are physiological anisocoria, tonic pupils, and traumatic pupillary abnormalities.
  - These abnormalities are not associated with other features of dysautonomia such as xerostomia, areflexia, diarrhea, hypotension, bradycardia, urinary retention, and erectile dysfunction.
- Tonic pupil is common among an otherwise normal population and is usually caused by damage to the ciliary ganglia by viral infection. The pupil reacts slowly to light and better to accommodation. Sometimes it is associated with loss of ankle reflexes and other DTRs due to involvement of dorsal root ganglia. Unlike normal pupil, tonic pupil reacts to pilocarpine due to denervation hypersensitivity.
- Light response of pupils in physiological anisocoria are normal (direct, indirect, and accommodation response).
- Patients do not usually volunteer information about old trauma to the eye, and the clinician must have a high index of suspicion.
- Mydriasis and isolated medial rectus weakness were concerning for oculomotor nerve palsy. In contrast, involvement of both medial and lateral recti, fluctuating ptosis, and normal level of consciousness could be explained by a unifying diagnosis of MG.

CASE 4.9: FLUCTUATING EOM WEAKNESS WITHOUT DIPLOPIA

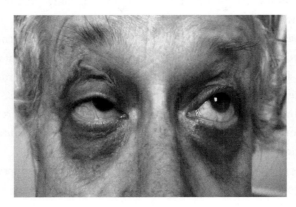

VIDEO 4.9

A 70 year-old-man presented with a 1-year history of variable right ptosis. His family noticed divergent eyes when he was tired, but he did not have diplopia. He had dysphagia and dysarthria. AChR antibody test was positive.

In MG, the lack of diplopia despite fatigable extraocular muscles (EOM) occurs in the following circumstances:

1. Complete ptosis
2. Negative serology
3. Monocular blindness (macular degeneration)
4. Negative repetitive nerve stimulation (RNS)
5. Thymoma

DIAGNOSIS

- His examination confirmed the presence of fatigable right ptosis and superior rectus weakness without diplopia.
- Chronic diffuse ophthalmoplegia, such as chronic progressive external ophthalmoplegia (CPEO) and oculopharyngeal muscular dystrophy (OPMD), are not typically associated with diplopia. The chronicity and gradual progression of these disorders allows the brain to suppress one image and thus avoid diplopia.
- Fluctuating binocular diplopia is an important feature of MG and results from fatigable weakness of one or more extraocular muscles. The diplopia can be horizontal, vertical, or oblique, depending on the affected muscle(s).
- However, diplopia is not reported by the patient if one eye does not produce an image due to complete ptosis, monocular blindness, long-standing strabismus, and so on.

CASE 4.10: OPHTHALMOPLEGIA WITH FREQUENT FALLS

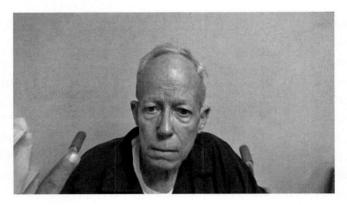

VIDEO 4.10

A 73-year-old-man presented with frequent falls.

The likely cause of the falls in this case is:

1. Neuropathy
2. Parkinson disease
3. Progressive supranuclear palsy (PSP)
4. Myasthenia gravis (MG)
5. Oculopharyngeal muscular dystrophy (OPMD)

DIAGNOSIS

- Ophthalmoplegia means paralysis of one or more extraocular muscle (EOM).
- There are several ways of classifying ophthalmoplegia:
  - Acute or chronic:
    - Acute ophthalmoplegia is usually associated with diplopia, unlike chronic ones.
  - External or internal:
    - Pupillary dilatation (internal ophthalmoplegia) is not a feature of MG but may be seen in compressive oculomotor palsy, and in presynaptic neuromuscular disorders.
    - External ophthalmoplegia is usually a feature of muscle disease (CPEO, OPMD), myasthenia, or non-compressive oculomotor palsy (diabetic 3rd cranial nerve palsy).
  - Supranuclear or infranuclear:
    - Supranuclear, as in PSP
    - Infranuclear, such as myopathies and neuromuscular junction disorders
- Doll's eye movement is preserved in the supranuclear type.
- The presented case showed the patient looking to the right as a reflex to the speaker's voice (second 16 of the recording). He could not do the same movement on command. This pattern is typically seen in supranuclear ophthalmoplegia.
- Progressive supranuclear palsy: neurodegenerative disease of the central nervous system (CNS) characterized by:
  - Impairment of vertical gaze (later becomes global gaze palsy) and axial rigidity leading to frequent falls.
  - Dysarthria, dysphagia, dementia, and emotional incontinence are common.
  - Rare blinking and facial dystonia.
  - Tau-positive filamentous inclusions intracellularly in specific anatomic areas are characteristic.
  - Other features of multiple system atrophy (MSA) may be evident, such as extrapyramidal symptoms.
- Diagnosis remains clinical and prognosis is poor.

CASE 4.11: DIPLOPIA AND TRICEPS FATIGABILITY

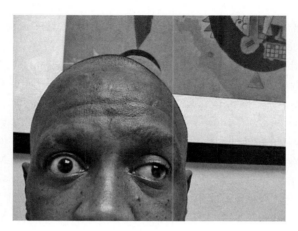

VIDEO 4.11

A 43-year-old man reported diplopia triggered by facing bright lights while driving. Sunglasses and prisms helped temporarily, but symptoms returned after a few months. He then developed difficulty doing bench presses. Examination is shown.

The most likely diagnosis is:

1. Internuclear ophthalmoplegia (INO)
2. Congenital myasthenic syndrome (CMS)
3. Chronic progressive external ophthalmoplegia (CPEO)
4. Myasthenia gravis (MG)
5. Oculopharyngeal muscular dystrophy (OPMD)

DIAGNOSIS

- Video showed fatigable ptosis and weakness of multiple EOMs and fatigable triceps.
- Triceps muscle is commonly involved in MG, especially in African Americans, and it rarely can be the presenting feature of the disease. Biceps are much less affected.
- Patients tend to modify their activities to avoid using the triceps for months or years before other muscles become affected and medical advice is sought.
- Triceps muscles may be strong in the beginning of resistance but fatigue easily; therefore, in every suspected myasthenic, triceps muscles should be tested for fatigue.
- None of the mentioned options causes fatigue of triceps, other than MG and CMS.
- Triceps weakness and fatigability may persist despite improvement of other muscles.

CASE 4.12: DROOPY EYELIDS AND FAINTING

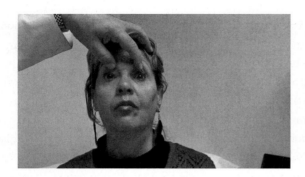

VIDEO 4.12

A 53-year-old woman presented with symptoms since age 23, consisting of droopy eyelids and impairment of night vision. She fainted one time and was taken to the emergency room. She was discharged from the hospital with a pacemaker. She had seven children who were all healthy. Myasthenia serology was negative, but she thought that pyridostigmine was helpful.

The most likely diagnosis is:

1. Oculopharyngeal muscular dystrophy (OPMD)
2. Congenital myasthenic syndrome (CMS)
3. Myasthenia gravis (MG)
4. Kearns-Sayre syndrome (KSS)
5. Myotonic dystrophy (MD)

DIAGNOSIS

- Video showed fixed ophthalmoplegia and bilateral ptosis. Night vision loss suggested retinitis pigmentosa, which was confirmed by fundoscopic examination. Syncope was due to heart block, which was not a feature of MG.
- The diagnosis of Kearns-Sayre syndrome (KSS) was made based on mitochondrial analysis on muscle tissue.
- Positive response to pyridostigmine is not specific.
- Cardiac conduction abnormalities are common in mitochondrial disorders and predict high mortality and morbidity.
- Early detection by regular monitoring is important to reduce chances of sudden death, as progression to high grade AV block is not predictable.
- Cardiac conduction abnormalities occur in 85% of patients with KSS and 10% of other mitochondrial disorders, mostly m.3243>G and m.8344A>G mutations.
- Other cardiac conduction defects, such as supraventricular arrhythmias, prolonged QT interval, and preexcitation syndromes, are all reported more in patients with mitochondrial disorders than in the general population.
- Different kinds of cardiomyopathies are reported in 40% of mitochondrial disorders.
- Cases of predominant cardiac involvement with minimal additional manifestations are reported in some mitochondrial mutations.

REFERENCE

Bates MGD, et al. Cardiac involvement in mitochondrial DNA disease: clinical spectrum, diagnosis, and management. *European Heart Journal.* 2012;33:3023–3033.

CASE 4.13: PTOSIS SINCE CHILDHOOD

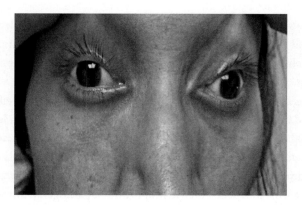

VIDEO 4.13

A 36-year-old-man presented with bilateral fixed ptosis since 10 years of age. Over the preceding 10 years, he developed mild dysphagia and proximal leg weakness. Examination revealed no sensory abnormalities, cardiac conduction problems, deafness, or visual impairment. Serum resting lactate and pyruvate were normal. Brain MRI was normal. EMG revealed mild myopathic features in the proximal leg muscles. Repetitive nerve stimulation (RNS) test was negative. CK level was normal. MG serology was negative. Muscle biopsy showed many ragged red fibers.

The next most useful diagnostic step is to send muscle tissue for:

1. Mitochondrial mutations
2. Muscle end plate analysis
3. PABPN1 mutation
4. Muscle microarray
5. Chromosomal analysis (karyotype)

DIAGNOSIS

- The video showed fixed and severe bilateral ptosis and ophthalmoplegia.
- Mitochondrial disorders are commonly seen in neuromuscular clinics as well as other subspecialty clinics due to their protean manifestations and the wide range of affected age groups.
- Mitochondria are bacteria that insinuated into the living human cell a billion years ago and have lived in it symbiotically, therefore losing their full independence.
- Mitochondrial DNA (mtDNA) contains only 37 genes. MtDNA encodes 13 of the 80 proteins that compose the respiratory chain. Nuclear DNA controls the remaining 99% of mitochondrial proteins.
- Phenotypic variation depends on the proportion of pathogenic mitochondria in the tissue. Heteroplasmy implies the presence of pathogenic and healthy mitochondria side by side in the same host. In a neuromuscular patient, the presence of multisystemic involvement such as seizures, deafness, neuropathy, myopathy, ophthalmoplegia, cardiomyopathy, and so on, should raise the possibility of mitochondrial disorders.
- Phenotype may change as the patient ages, due to mitotic segregation of pathogenic mitochondria during cell division.
- Mitochondrial DNA mutations are maternally inherited, which prevents male to male transmission. Pedigree analysis can be very helpful.

Neuromuscular mitochondrial disorders:

- mtDNA mutations:
  - mtDNA deletions:
    - Kearns-Sayre syndrome
    - Chronic progressive external ophthalmoplegia
  - Point mutations:
    - Myoclonic epilepsy, lactic acidosis, and strokes (MELAS)
    - Myoclonic epilepsy and ragged red fibers (MERRF)
    - Neuropathy, ataxia, and retinitis pigmentosa (NARP)
    - Mitochondrial myopathies: exercise intolerance, rhabdomyolysis, and myalgia
- Nuclear DNA (nDNA) mutations:
  - Mitochondrial neurogastrointestinal encephalopathy (MNGIE)
  - ANT1 mutations
  - POLG mutations:
    - AD or AR CPEO
    - SANDO
    - MIRAS
  - Twinkle mutations

CASE 4.14: MUSCLE STIFFNESS AND WEIGHT LOSS

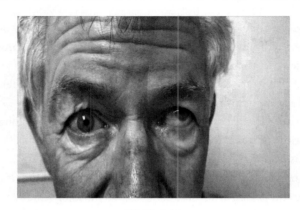

VIDEO 4.14

A 62-year-old-man developed severe intermittent stiffness of the back and leg muscles (triggered by cold), diplopia, progressive hearing loss, and intermittent severe vertigo. He also developed photophobia, headache, and irritability. He had nasopharyngeal carcinoma treated with radiation 3 years earlier. Symptoms responded well to diazepam. EMG showed no myotonia or spontaneous motor unit discharges. Repetitive nerve stimulation was normal. AChR antibody titer was negative. Sodium channel (SC4A) mutation was negative. GAD antibodies titer was more than 30 nU/ml.

The most likely diagnosis is:

1. Progressive encephalomyelitis rigidity and myoclonus (PERM)
2. Neuromyotonia
3. Paramyotonia congenita
4. Myasthenia gravis
5. None of the above

DIAGNOSIS

- Paraneoplastic neuromuscular syndromes may present individually or in combinations.
- Some of these syndromes are not difficult to diagnose, such as progressive cerebellar ataxia in a patient with small cell lung cancer or lymphoma.
- Diagnostic difficulties arise when the cancer is not diagnosed or when the symptoms are vague and diffuse, as in this case.
- Cold-sensitive muscle stiffness is typically seen in paramyotonia congenita, which is not a paraneoplastic syndrome. However, the age of the patient and EOM abnormality were atypical for this disorder.
- Stiff person syndrome (SPS) was a strong possibility. Axial stiffness is not as prominent in paraneoplastic stiff person syndrome compared to the idiopathic syndrome.
- The patient responded well to diazepam, which supported the diagnosis of SPS.
- The displayed ophthalmoplegia was difficult to reconcile with a typical case of SPS.
- Lambert-Eaton myasthenic syndrome (LEMS), which may occur on a paraneoplastic basis, can have abnormality of extraocular motility. However, eye findings are typically less prominent than in MG, and LEMS patients more typically present with proximal weakness and autonomic symptoms and their examination shows facilitation of strength and reflexes with exercise. In this case, voltage-gated calcium channels antibodies were negative, RNS was normal, and there was no facilitation of compound muscle action potential (CMAP) amplitudes with exercise.
- The constellation of vertigo, deafness, headache, photophobia, and the rapid progression in a patient with cancer suggested paraneoplastic brain stem encephalitis. Elevated CSF protein supported that conclusion. Negative brain MRI may be due to the subtle nature of the inflammation.
- SPS with encephalitis is reported with some malignancies and is associated with increased antibodies to anti-amphiphysin.
- Progressive encephalomyelitic rigidity and myoclonus (PERM):
  - A variant of SPS that is associated with ophthalmoplegia, nystagmus, myoclonus, hearing loss, vertigo, and dysautonomia
  - Reported with lymphoma
  - Death within 4 years is common in most cases

REFERENCE

Wessig C, Klein R, Schneider MF, Toyka KV, Naumann M, Sommer C. Neuropathology and binding studies in anti-amphiphysin-associated stiff-person syndrome. *Neurology*. 2003;61(2):195.

CASE 4.15: FAMILIAL PTOSIS

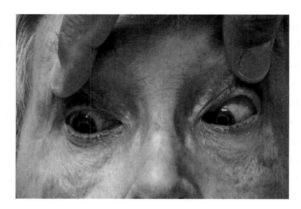

VIDEO 4.15

A 77-year-old-woman presented with a 20-year history of droopy eyelids and dysphagia. She had a brother and a sister with the same. She had mild proximal weakness. CK level was 200 U/L and EMG was myopathic.

This disorder is due to a mutation of:

1. Polyadenylate binding protein nuclear 1 (PABPN1)
2. mtDNA
3. Rapsyn gene
4. Na channel gene
5. Ca channel gene

CASE 5.1: MUSCLE STIFFNESS AND SYNCOPE

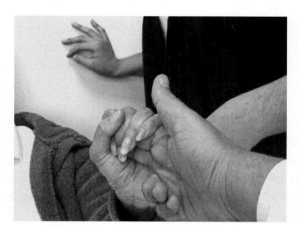

VIDEO 5.1

A 65-year-old-woman presented to the emergency room twice during a year due to syncope. She was found to have complete heart block and had a pacemaker. Her creatine kinase (CK) level was 800 U/L with normal echocardiogram and thallium stress test. She had no family history of muscle disease. Her father had cataract surgery at age 50 years.

The history and examination provide findings typically seen in:

1. Myotonia congenita
2. Myotonic dystrophy
3. Paramyotonia congenita
4. Schwartz-Jampel syndrome
5. Anderson Tawil syndrome

DIAGNOSIS

The slow relaxation phase that improves with repeated testing (warming-up phenomenon) is typically seen in myotonia. The frontal baldness and facial weakness suggest myotonic dystrophy. Cataract in her father with minimal muscular symptoms and more severe symptoms in the patient suggest anticipation. Syncope due to heart block is common in myotonic dystrophy.

- Myotonic dystrophy:
  - Myotonic dystrophy is the most common inherited neuromuscular disorder (13.5/100,000 live births).
  - It is an autosomal dominant (AD) disease due to mutation of myotonic dystrophy protein kinase (DMPK) gene located in the non-coding region of the gene.
  - Severity correlates with CTG repeat number:
    - 50–150 repeats: mild disease
    - 100–1,000 repeats: moderate disease
    - More than 1,000 repeats: severe
  - Earlier and more severe symptoms in successive generations are characteristic of the disease, and this is called "anticipation."
    - Anticipation is explained by successive prolongation of the CTG repeat expansion due to instability of the gene.
    - The number of repeats varies from one tissue to another.
    - Loss of DMPK function is associated with altered Ca^{++} homeostasis. The exact molecular mechanism by which the genotype produces phenotype is not clear.
- Clinical features:
  - Myotonia: it correlates with CTG repeats
  - Ptosis and facial weakness
    - No ophthalmoplegia
  - Proximal and distal weakness
  - Apathy and mental retardation
  - Hypersomnia
  - Hypogonadism, hypothyroidism, and diabetes mellitus
  - Cardiac abnormalities
  - Tachyarrhythmia
  - Atrial flutter and fibrillation
  - Sudden death
  - Cardiomyopathy
    - Annual EKG is indicated and cardiac intervention is needed if there is a progressive prolongation of PR interval or QRS duration.
  - Dysphagia and megacolon
  - Medications to be avoided: tricyclic antidepressants, beta blockers, anti-arrhythmics

CASE 5.2: FACIAL WEAKNESS AND ELEVATED CSF PROTEIN

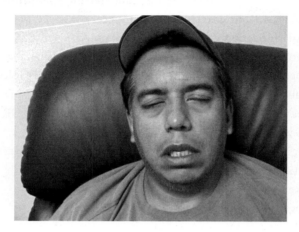

VIDEO 5.2

A 30-year-old man presented with a 2-week history of acute tingling of the feet and hands, difficulty raising his arms, and a 1-week history of slurring of speech and dryness of the eyes. He had no preceding fever. Cerebrospinal fluid (CSF) protein was 280 mg/ml, and the nerve conduction study (NCS) revealed prolonged F responses and distal latencies with motor slowing of several nerves in all extremities.

Bilateral facial palsy is a feature of:

1. Guillain-Barré syndrome (GBS)
2. Sarcoidosis
3. Lyme disease
4. Bilateral Bell palsy
5. All of the above

DIAGNOSIS

- Bilateral facial nerve palsy is defined as a simultaneous or sequential weakness of both sides of the face. It complicates 0.3%–2% of facial paralysis.
- Facial onset GBS is one of several clinical variants of GBS.
  - It is symmetric and occurs early, along with extremities weakness. It should be noted that asymmetric facial diplegia may occur later in the disease while other motor symptoms are stable or improving.
  - 86% of cases are preceded by upper respiratory tract infection (URTI) by 2–4 weeks.
  - Age: 23–65 years.
  - Facial diplegia progresses over 4 weeks. It is important to close eyes with eye patches or scotch tape at bedtime to avoid exposure keratitis.
  - Feet numbness
  - Mild or no weakness
  - Areflexia
  - CSF albumino-cytologic dissociation
  - Demyelination noted in NCS in 64% of patients.
- Causes of facial diplegia:
  - Guillain-Barré syndrome
  - HIV infection: may occur before seroconversion
  - Sarcoidosis
  - Melkersson syndrome
  - Hereditary: Möbius syndrome and congenital facial paresis
  - Leprosy
  - An-α-lipoproteinemia (Tangier)
  - Lyme disease
  - Other peripheral causes:
    - Motor neuron disorders such as Kennedy disease
    - Myasthenia gravis (MG)
    - Myopathies: myotonic dystrophy, facioscapulohumeral muscular dystrophy (FSHD), inclusion body myositis (IBM)
- Other regional variants of GBS:
  - Miller-Fisher Syndrome
  - Pharyngeal-cervical-brachial variants
  - Paraparetic variant
  - Acute sensory polyneuropathy
  - Acute autonomic neuropathy

REFERENCE

Susuki K, Koga M, Hirata K, Isogai E, Yuki N. A Guillain-Barré syndrome variant with prominent facial diplegia. *J Neurol.* 2009 Nov;256(11):1899–1905. doi:10.1007/s00415-009-5254-8. Epub 2009 Jul 25.

CASE 5.3: RESOLUTION OF FACIAL WEAKNESS

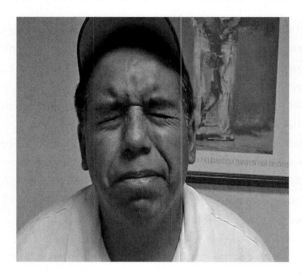

VIDEO 5.3

The patient was treated with intravenous immunoglobulin (IVIG) 1 gm/kg of body weight every day for two days. This examination was done a month later.

Which of the following treatments is (are) proven to be affective first line therapy in GBS?

1. Intravenous gammaglobulin
2. Intravenous steroids
3. Plasmapheresis
4. Rituximab
5. Azathioprine

DIAGNOSIS

- Intravenous (IV) steroids did not beat the placebo in treatment of GBS; some treated patients became worse. Adding IV steroids to IVIG did not offer benefit in clinical trials.
- IVIG and therapeutic plasma exchange (TPE) are equally effective and have comparable side effects profiles.
  - The main IVIG complications are headache, myalgia, renal impairment, and deep vein thrombosis (DVT).
  - The main side effects of TPE are hypotension, hypocalcaemia, and vascular access–related complications such as infection, obstruction, and bleeding.
- TPE after IVIG does not make sense, and IVIG after TPE does not offer benefit.
- Patients with congestive cardiac failure (CCF) are more suitable for TPE, while patients with infection are more suitable for IVIG.
- TPE onset is shorter than IVIG but vascular access is inhibitory.
- With the introduction of smaller machines and outpatient availability and the ease of vascular access, TPE is being used more widely than before.
- Subcutaneous immunoglobulin (SCIg) is emerging as an alternative to IVIG but clinical trials are lacking so far.
- While all GBS patients need to be monitored closely in order to detect bulbar involvement early, not every GBS patient has to be treated. Treatment is indicated in:
  - Patients with ambulation problems
  - Patients seen within 6 weeks of the onset of symptoms
- Milder cases and cases seen later in the disease course are not generally treated.
- Dosage:
  - TPE: 250 ml/kg/bwt over 10–14 days. It usually translates to 5-6 (one plasma volume per session) exchanges over two weeks.
  - IVIG 2 gm/kg/bwt over 2–5 days.
- Improvement is noted in 1–3 weeks after treatment.
- Chronic inflammatory demyelinating polyneuropathy (CIDP) may present acutely and therefore can be confused with GBS. Ten percent of treated GBS patients relapse within weeks. In these cases, CIDP should be considered.

CASE 5.4: CARPOPEDAL SPASMS

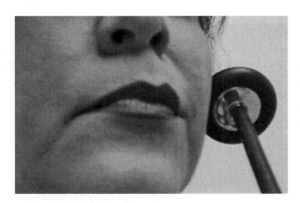

VIDEO 5.4

A 27-year-old woman had developed tingling of the hands and feet with intermittent spontaneous painful spasms of the fingers and toes, facial twitching, and nervousness over the preceding 6 months. Electromyogram (EMG) revealed many doublets.

These symptoms and signs suggest:

1. Hypercalcemia
2. Hypocalcemia
3. Tetanus
4. Myokymia
5. Neuromyotonia

DIAGNOSIS

- Examination showed weakness of the left face that involved both volitional and emotional components and involving the upper and lower parts of the face.
- Facial palsy is a common presentation to the neuromuscular clinics.
- The facial muscles are supplied by the facial nerves that emerge from the pontomedullary junction and enter the face through the parotid glands.
- Chorda tympani carries taste sensation to the anterior two-thirds of the tongue and joins the facial nerve later in the course. It also carries parasympathetic supply to the lacrimal and salivary glands except parotids. The smallest muscle in the body (the stapedius) is supplied by a branch of facial nerve, and it tenses and relaxes the tympanic membrane during transmission of air vibrations to produce clear distinction of sound.
- Facial nerve may be affected by myopathies (FSHD, IBM, etc.), polyneuropathies (CIDP, FAN), mononeuropathies (Bell palsy, sarcoidosis), MG, brain stem pathology (ischemic, glioma), and cerebral pathology (infarction, etc.).
- The face is bilaterally innervated and therefore central facial weakness saves the upper part of the face, while peripheral facial palsy as in Bell palsy leads to loss of upper and lower facial strength.
- Bell palsy is an acute peripheral facial paralysis due to viral invasion of the nerve at the stylomastoid canal. HSV1 is the most common proven infection, followed by herpes zoster activation, CMV, and EBV.
- Acute retroauricular pain is followed by facial palsy, loss of taste of the anterior two-thirds of the tongue, hyperacusis, and dry eyes.
- Onset occurs over a day or two, maximum weakness in 3 weeks, and recovery in 6 months.
- Recurrence occurs in 7% of cases and a second recurrence in 2%.
- Prednisone 60–80 mg a day for a week is shown to reduce risk of unfavorable recovery if given early in the course of the disease.
- Antiviral therapy is no routinely needed as double blind clinical trials did not favor them.

CASE 5.6: FACIAL WEAKNESS AFTER DIVORCE

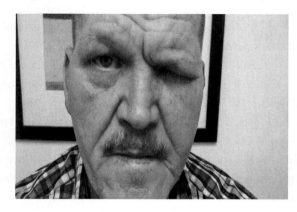

VIDEO 5.6

A 55-year-old man presented with a history of metastatic prostate cancer and a recent divorce and loss of his job. He suddenly could not open his left eye and developed frontal headache with no sensory symptoms. Examination a month later is shown. Symptoms resolved with intramuscular facial normal saline injection.

The features that suggest non-organic weakness in this case are:

1. Preservation of the nasolabial fold
2. Lack of facial weakness
3. Exaggerated wrinkles and facial folds in the affected side
4. Concurrent stress
5. All of the above

DIAGNOSIS

- His examination showed exaggeration of the upper facial folds and no objective facial weakness. There was no atrophy of the nasolabial fold (NLF).
- Facial weakness is often a manifestation of functional disorders and malingering since it can be easily mimicked. However, it is not difficult for a neurologist to recognize functional facial weakness.
- The elevation of the ipsilateral eyebrow and the closure of the ipsilateral eye are very suggestive of a functional overlay.
- Exaggeration of forehead wrinkles and preservation of the NLF are also suggestive of a non-organic cause. In Bell palsy, it is hard to close the affected eye, and the NLF becomes flat within a few days.
- Underlying stress may not be easy to figure out.
- Despite chronicity, atrophy does not occur and symptoms improve with distraction.
- Many patients respond to treatment with a placebo.

CASE 5.7: FACIAL ASYMMETRY AFTER A HURRICANE

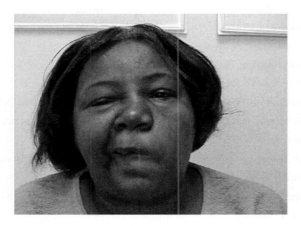

VIDEO 5.7

A 65-year-old woman relocated to Houston after losing her house and job due to Hurricane Katrina. She developed frequent sustained painful right facial muscle spasms every time she saw her friends who lived in the same area. The condition always resolved with prayer.

The following facts support a functional rather than organic hemifacial spasms:

1. They are sustained.
2. They are painful.
3. They are associated with profound speech abnormality.
4. They are worsened by stress.
5. They are improved by prayer.

DIAGNOSIS

- There was no facial weakness, but her voice changed during the spasms. Chvostek sign was negative.
- Stress may be associated with a wide spectrum of clinical manifestations; some of them are difficult to differentiate from their organic counterparts.
- Rarely is the source of stress apparent, but when it is, the diagnosis is facilitated.
- Symptoms are usually not typical for any recognized neurological presentation.
- It is important to differentiate between:
  - Conversion: stress is converted into acute somatic symptoms such as weakness or numbness, usually in young females.
  - Somatization: stress is converted into chronic multiple somatic symptoms usually in middle-aged females.
  - Factitious disorder: symptoms are induced by administration of pharmacologically active substances such as insulin injections to produce hypoglycemia.
  - Malingering: fabrication of symptoms.
    - The first three are involuntary and the fourth is a conscious falsification.
- While psychogenic symptoms typically improve with prayer and get worse with stress, this does not exclude organicity as many organic symptoms improve with these measures, too.

CASE 5.8: COULD NEVER BLOW A BALLOON

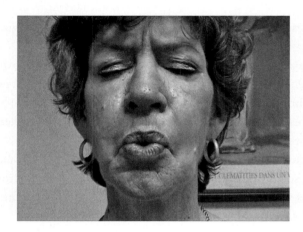

VIDEO 5.8

A 63-year-old woman presented with a 20-year history of inability to stand on her heels and a 10-year history of inability to stand from a deep chair and difficulty raising her arms. She could never blow a balloon. Her examination is shown.

The combination of facial weakness, foot drop, and scapular winging that evolves over years is very typical of FSHD.

What do the identified structures in Figure 5.8.1 (arrows) represent?

1. Scapulae
2. Hypertrophied trapezius
3. Levator scapulae
4. Fat pad
5. Sternocleidomastoid

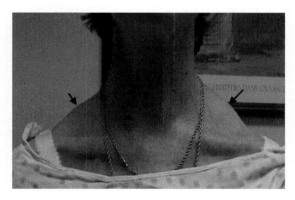

FIGURE 5.8.1 A patient with FSHD.

DIAGNOSIS

- Facial weakness is frequently the first sign of FSHD, although it is not usually noticed by patients but by their friends and family members.
- Retrospectively, many patients give a history of difficulty with blowing balloons, using straws, and whistling for years before the diagnosis. Patients cannot pucker lips on exam. Labial dysarthria may occur. Transverse smile is common.
- Inability to close eyes completely during sleep may cause exposure keratitis. Patching the eyes during sleep may be necessary.
- Facial involvement occurs in 95% of cases. In the remaining 5% the face is spared.
  - These are usually of late onset and are associated with small deletions.
- In 7% of cases, facial involvement is predominant and scapuloperoneal weakness is only found in the examination.
- Facial weakness is common in IBM and myotonic dystrophy. Dysphagia and true proximal weakness are rare in FSHD.
- The inability to abduct arms is not due to weakness of the arm abductor muscles but due to instability of the scapulae, which ascend and rotate during arms abduction, forming the arrowed prominences.

CASE 5.9: A PENALTY FOR FACIAL LIFT

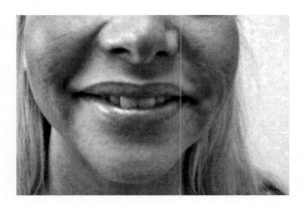

VIDEO 5.9

A 45-year-old woman had bilateral transoral cheek implantation, facelift, and rhinoplasty 3 months earlier. She could not pucker her upper lip or whistle since surgery. There was no weakness in the rest of the face and her facial sensation was normal. EMG revealed denervation of the upper lip only.

The mentioned findings suggest an injury to the following branches of the facial nerve:

1. Main trunk
2. Marginal branches
3. Buccal branches
4. Frontal branches
5. Cervical branches

DIAGNOSIS

- Rhytidectomy (facelift) is the 6th most common plastic surgery in the United States and each facelift costs $10,000 on average.
- Nerve injury is one of the most common complications. The facial and greater auricular nerves are the most commonly affected.
- Many cases recover spontaneously within a few months.
- Permanent motor nerve paralysis occurs at a rate of 0.5%–2.6%.
  - The marginal branch is most commonly injured, followed by frontal and buccal branches. In this case the buccal branches were severed.
- Pseudoparalysis of the marginal mandibular nerve due to cervical branch injury can be distinguished from true marginal mandibular injury by the fact that the patient will be able to evert the lower lip because of a functioning mentalis muscle.
- The prevalence of cervical branch injury in facelifts is reported at 1.7%.
- Sensory nerve injuries are more common, with great auricular nerve injury reported in up to 7% of cases.

CASE 5.10: WEAKNESS OF FACE AND FINGERS

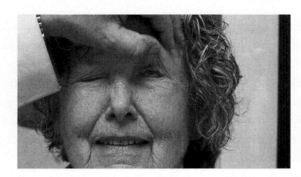

VIDEO 5.10

A 77-year-old woman reported a 5-year history of difficulty climbing stairs and dysphagia. Creatine kinase (CK) was 190 IU/L, and the EMG revealed many short-duration polyphasic units in the proximal leg muscles and finger flexors.

Muscle biopsy in this disease is not expected to show:

1. Endomysial inflammation
2. Cytoplasmic inclusion bodies
3. Red-rimmed vacuoles
4. Denervated fibers
5. Perifascicular atrophy

DIAGNOSIS

- The video revealed facial weakness, finger flexors weakness, and proximal leg weakness.
- Inclusion body myositis is the most common myopathy after age 50 years. It is more common in males.
- While a typical picture is that of chronic progressive weakness of quadriceps (more than iliopsoas), finger flexors, and biceps (more than deltoids) and dysphagia, phenotypic variations are well reported.
- In this case, the quadriceps muscles were not clinically affected.
- Dysphagia occurs in two-thirds of cases.
- Unlike polymyositis and dermatomyositis, facial weakness occurs in one-third of cases, although it is often discovered during examination and the patient does not complain about it. It can be so severe that eyes cannot be kept closed during sleep, which may lead to exposure keratitis.
- Typical pathological findings include:
  - Chronic myopathic changes (variation of fiber size and shape, necrotic and phagocytic fibers, spit fibers, patchy loss of oxidative activity, increased connective tissue, etc.).
  - Endomysial inflammation with invasion of non-necrotic fibers with mononuclear inflammatory cells.
  - Red-rimmed vacuoles and eosinophilic cytoplasmic inclusion bodies.
  - Nuclear inclusion bodies seen under electron microscope (EM).
  - Congophilic material usually adjacent to the vacuoles.
  - Denervated fibers.
    - Perifascicular atrophy is not a feature of IBM. It is typically seen in dermatomyositis.

CASE 5.11: NASAL SPEECH

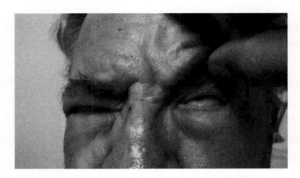

VIDEO 5.11

A 65-year-old man presented with a 3-month history of nasal speech and regurgitation of water through the nose.

Facial weakness and nasal speech are typically seen in:

1. Myasthenia gravis (MG)
2. Lambert-Eaton myasthenic syndrome (LEMS)
3. Inclusion body myositis (IBM)
4. Facioscapulohumeral muscular dystrophy (FSMD)
5. Chronic inflammatory demyelinating polyneuropathy (CIDP)

DIAGNOSIS

- The video revealed facial weakness and nasal speech.
- Facial weakness is common in MG and several myopathies like IBM and myotonic dystrophy.
- LEMS usually presents with proximal weakness mimicking myopathy. Facial weakness is rare.
- Guillain-Barré syndrome may lead to facial diplegia.
- Palate weakness, causing nasal speech and regurgitation of food through nose, is not commonly seen in any of the mentioned possibilities except MG.
- The most common causes of nasal speech are local factors such as adenoids, deviated septum, and allergic rhinitis. Neurologic causes are rare and include MG, poliomyelitis, and diphtheria.

CASE 5.12: FACIAL TWITCHING

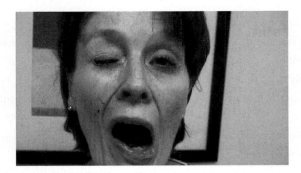

VIDEO 5.12

A 48-year-old woman had right Bell palsy 2 years earlier from which she recovered, except for the finding that is shown in the video.

The eye blinking is due to:

1. Viral reactivation
2. Synkinesis of facial nerve
3. Is not related to Bell palsy
4. Is reversible most of the time

DIAGNOSIS

- Facial synkinesis is a common complication of Bell palsy.
- During nerve regeneration, nerve misdirected wiring may occur, leading to misconnection of different nerve fibers that are intended for different functions.
- It is more likely to happen in severe cases.
- Synkinesis is manifested during the recovery process, usually months after the initial insult.
- The most common symptoms of facial synkinesis are:
  - Eye closure with volitional contraction of mouth muscles
    - This patient demonstrated an involuntary blinking of the right eye whenever she opened her mouth.
  - Facial movements with volitional eye closure
  - Neck tightness (platysmal contraction) with volitional smiling
  - Hyper-lacrimation (also called Crocodile Tears)
    - A case where eating or just thinking of food provokes excessive lacrimation: this has been attributed to neural synkinesis between branches to the salivary glands and the lacrimal glands.
    - The condition is chronic and may be helped by Botulinum toxin injections to the lacrimal glands.

CASE 5.13: INABILITY TO SING AND KISS

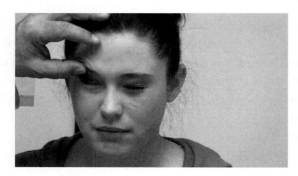

VIDEO 5.13

A 17-year-old girl presented with a 1-year history of inability to sing in church because her voice faded soon after she began singing. Binding AChR antibody titer was 403 nmol/L.

Such a very high AChR antibody titer:

1. Indicates a poor prognosis
2. Indicates severe disease
3. Is associated with high risk of generalization of MG
4. Is associated with thymoma
5. Confirms the diagnosis of MG

DIAGNOSIS

- The video showed upper and lower facial weakness.
- Absolute titer of AChR binding antibodies does not correlate with severity of MG in the general population, although in individual patients, improvement is often seen with reduction in titer by more than 50%.
  - These antibodies are positive in 80%–90% of generalized and 50%–70% of ocular MG.
  - False positive rarely occurs in:
    - Lambert-Eaton syndrome
    - Graft vs. host disease
    - Autoimmune hepatitis
    - Healthy relatives of patients with myasthenia
    - Patients with thymoma
    - Lung cancer
    - Motor neuron disease
    - Snake venom poisoning
- There is no difference in phenotype or responsiveness to treatment between seronegative and seropositive individuals (regardless of the titer).
- Antibodies may not even decline with treatment, despite good clinical response.
- Seroconversion occurs in 20% of cases within a year; therefore, repeating the test in negative cases is advised.
- Anti-ACh receptor blocking and modulating antibodies are reported in 5% of AChR binding antibody cases. They may be useful if the binding antibodies are negative. This test is reported on a percentage basis and should be considered significant only when present at a high percentile. Minimally positive test results in normal patients are not uncommon.
- Anti-ACh blocking antibodies are highly specific. False positives are only rarely reported in LEMS and in patients exposed to curare-like drugs. These are essentially never present in isolation. Accordingly, these are not used as a screening test for MG, and their only practical role is to aid in the identification of a potentially false-positive result.
- Other than confirming the diagnosis, AChR antibody titer does not have a prognostic value, correlates with severity, or predicts thymoma.

CASE 5.14: CROOKED SMILE SINCE CHILDHOOD

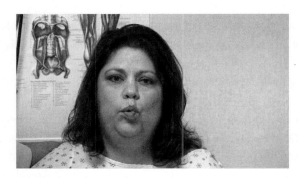

VIDEO 5.14

A 42-year-old woman presented with a history of diabetes mellitus and hypertension; she was noticed to have a crooked smile since the age of 12 years. Gradually she noticed difficulty raising her arms and pain in the upper back. She had normal deep tendon reflexes (DTRs), sensation, feet extensors, hearing, and vision. Physical findings are shown. She had one child and four siblings. There was no family history of a neurological illness.

The most likely cause of facial weakness in this case is:

1. Facial nerve palsy
2. Facioscapulohumeral muscular dystrophy (FSHD)
3. Scapuloperoneal syndrome
4. Congenital facial weakness
5. Demyelinating neuropathy

DIAGNOSIS

- Asymmetrical facial weakness, scapular winging, inverted axillary folds, and proximal leg weakness since age 12 are very suggestive of FSHD. Mutation analysis confirmed deletion of D4Z4 at 4q35.
- It is the second most prevalent form of muscular dystrophy after DMD with prevalence of 5/100,000.
- Asymmetry in FSHD is so striking that some patients are diagnosed with facial nerve palsy. Asymmetrical foot drop is common.
- It is an autosomal dominant disease but 30% of cases are caused by de novo mutation.
- The genotype-phenotype relationship is far from being understood. Interestingly, a toxic gain of function of DUX4 is found to play a role. This is the first time where a "junk DNA" is found to reanimate and cause disease.
- Life span is normal. Twenty percent of patients eventually require a wheelchair and 1% artificial ventilation.

REFERENCE

Lemmers, RJ, et al. A unifying genetic model for FSHD. *Science*. 2010 Sep 24;1650–1653.

CHAPTER 6

TONGUE SIGNS

CASE 6.1: SLURRED SPEECH AND TROUBLE SWALLOWING

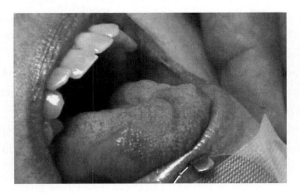

VIDEO 6.1

A 53-year-old woman presented with a 3-month history of slurring of speech and excessive drooling. She was suspected of having a stroke. Brain magnetic resonance imaging (MRI) was normal. She developed dysphagia a month later. Examination demonstrated key physical and neurophysiological findings. She had no weakness in the extremities.

The following are bad prognostic signs in this disease:

1. Onset in the legs
2. Bulbar onset
3. Spasticity
4. Old age
5. Female gender

DIAGNOSIS

- The examination showed atrophy and fasciculations of the tongue with jaw hyperreflexia, and tongue electromyogram (EMG) revealed fast firing motor units in the background.
- A third of ALS patients present with dysarthria and, to a lesser extent, dysphagia. The appearance of dysphagia before dysarthria is not typical of ALS.
- Early in the course of the disease and when clinical findings are confined to the bulbar muscles, diagnosis of ALS may be difficult, in particular if upper motor neuron (UMN) symptoms are predominant.
- Tongue fasciculations and jaw hyperreflexia are important clues to bulbar ALS, but when the lesion is confined to the UMN (PLS picture), confirmation of the diagnosis remains difficult.
- Bulbar onset occurs more in females, and it carries a worse prognosis than extremities onset ALS.
- Hypersialosis is common and may disturb swallowing further. If anticholinergic drugs fail, botulinum toxin injection to the salivary glands can be effective.
- Pseudobulbar affect (a tendency to laugh or cry with minimal provocation and with no emotional component) is common in bulbar ALS and is attributed to a UMN lesion and may respond well to tricyclic antidepressants or dextromethorphan/quinidine.
- Trials of riluzole showed that this medicine works better in bulbar onset ALS.
- The main differential diagnosis of bulbar palsy is myasthenia gravis, and more so, Musk Ab associated myasthenia gravis (MG). Therefore, AChR antibody titer should be checked and, if negative, Musk Ab titer.
- It is important to monitor pulmonary function tests (PFTs) since early institution of BiPAP is shown to improve quality of life and may prolong survival.
- Monitoring of swallowing is essential, and early PEG placement improves morbidity.
- Chronic lower motor neuron (LMN) bulbar palsy should raise the possibility of Kennedy disease, and one needs to examine breasts for gynecomastia and obtain mutation analysis for androgen receptors.
- Ptosis and ophthalmoplegia do not occur in bulbar ALS.
- Bulbar onset and old age are bad prognostic signs in ALS.

CASE 6.2: CHOKING WITH SALIVA

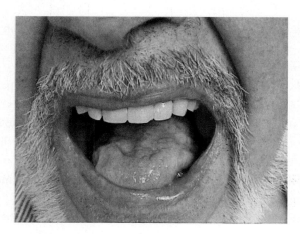

VIDEO 6.2

A 65-year-old man presented with a 6-month history of difficulty lifting his head for a long time. Two months later he developed slurring of speech, especially at night, and excessive salivation and choking. He lost 10 pounds. In addition to what is shown in the video, there was hyperreflexia of the jaw jerk and deep tendon reflexes in the upper and lower extremities. EMG revealed denervation of the tongue, neck extensors, and upper extremities proximally and distally. The thoracic paraspinal muscles and the leg muscles were not denervated.

This patient qualifies for which diagnosis, according to modified El Escorial Criteria?

1. Clinically definite ALS
2. Clinically probable ALS
3. Clinically probable-lab supported ALS
4. Possible ALS
5. No ALS

DIAGNOSIS

- The video revealed weak neck extensors, atrophy, and fasciculation of the tongue and dysarthria.
- There are several sets of ALS diagnostic criteria.
- In 1990, the World Federation of Neurology met in El Escorial in Spain and set diagnostic criteria for ALS that were mainly intended for research purposes. These criteria were modified 8 years later in order to allow more subjects to be enrolled in clinical trials. El Escorial Criteria (EEC) are the gold standard of ALS diagnosis, but the lack of sensitivity continues to stimulate experts to modify them.
- It is estimated that 25% of patients with progressive upper and lower motor neuron lesions proven at autopsy never met EEC.
- EEC do not capture those restricted variants such as primary lateral sclerosis (PLS), progressive muscular atrophy (PMA), and pseudobulbar palsy (PBP) that may never generalize.
- The following are the modified EEC criteria for the diagnosis of ALS. All require progressive course and exclusion of other causes by appropriate imaging and neurophysiological tests.
  - Clinically definite ALS: clinical evidence of UMN and LMN lesion in three regions
  - Clinically probable ALS: clinical evidence of UMN and LMN lesion in two regions and some UMN rostral to the LMN signs
  - Clinically probable–lab supported ALS: clinical evidence of UMN and LMN lesions in one region or clinical UMN signs in one region and EMG evidence of LMN in at least two limbs
  - Possible ALS: signs of UMN and LMN lesions in one region only or UMN signs in two or more regions
- The regions are: bulbar, cervical, thoracic, and lumbar.
- LMN evidence of denervation, according to El Escorial Criteria, is only fibrillations. (Awaji criteria allow for fasciculations.)
- This case qualified for clinically probable ALS. There was evidence of upper and lower motor neuron signs in the bulbar and cervical regions only.

CASE 6.3: JUST A LISP

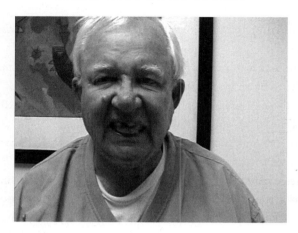

VIDEO 6.3

A 70-year-old man presented with a 6-month history of a "lisp," noted by his friends, that became worse the more he spoke. There was no diplopia, ptosis, dysphagia, muscle wasting, or extremities weakness. Since he was stressed, it was considered psychogenic. AChR antibody titer was high and the lingual dysarthria responded to steroids.

Lingual dysarthria can be a feature of:

1. Myasthenia gravis (MG)
2. Amyotrophic lateral sclerosis (ALS)
3. Hypoglossal neuropathy
4. Hysteria
5. Lambert-Eaton myasthenic syndrome (LEMS)

DIAGNOSIS

- The tongue consists of four pairs of extrinsic and four pairs of intrinsic muscles. Tongue movement is served by the hypoglossal nerve.
- Tongue weakness is a feature of several neuromuscular disorders. It may present as dysarthria or inability to move food in the mouth properly.
- These include muscle diseases (polymyositis), nerve diseases (GBS), neuromuscular junction (NMJ) disorders (MG, LEMS, botulism), motor neuron disease (ALS, Kennedy disease), and mitochondrial disorders like SANDO (sensory ataxia, neuropathy dysarthria, ophthalmoplegia).
- Bulbar weakness without prominent ocular symptoms is not unusual in MG. As a matter of fact, it is a common manifestation of MuSK antibodies associated MG, where atrophy of the tongue and face may lead to diagnostic confusion with bulbar onset ALS. Even tongue fasciculations are reported in MuSK antibodies associated MG.
- Fatigability of dysarthria (worsening with speech) is more typically seen in MG.
- In MG, the tip of the tongue is often affected early, leading to a "lisp"; in ALS, the bulk of the tongue is affected, leading to a "heavy tongue" like the tongue of an intoxicated person.
- Cerebellar dysarthria is irregular. The patient cannot count fast with regular intervals and consistent volume.

CASE 6.4: TONGUE PROTRUSIONS

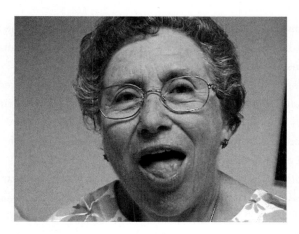

VIDEO 6.4

A 73-year-old woman presented with a 2-year history of abnormal tongue movement. There was no family history of a similar disorder. She had chronic nausea treated with metoclopramide for several months before these symptoms started.

The following drugs can cause this syndrome:

1. Metoclopramide
2. Hydrochlorothiazide
3. Promethazine
4. Tetracycline
5. Steroids

DIAGNOSIS

- The video showed involuntary painless repetitive protrusion of the tongue, which was alleviated by touching her face with her hand. There was no abnormal movement of the other facial muscles.
- Patients with oromandibular dystonia (OMD) are sometimes referred to neuromuscular (NM) clinics due to lingual dysarthria, dysphagia, choking, and weight loss that lead to suspicion of an NM disorder such as ALS or MG.
- Involuntary tongue protrusion in dystonia is usually associated with mouth opening and contraction of cervical muscles.
- The tongue in this syndrome is not weak or atrophied, and it is not fatigable.
- Oculogyric crisis, if it happens, can be easily differentiated from weak extraocular muscles (EOM) of MG.
- OMD is usually alleviated with sensory tricks such as touching the face.
- Like tardive dyskinesia, tardive dystonia can be produced by prolonged administration of drugs that block dopamine, such as phenothiazine and metoclopramide.
- OMD can also be produced by neurodegenerative disorders, but it is usually idiopathic.
- Botulinum toxin injection into genioglossus that protrudes the tongue usually works and does not cause swallowing problems.

CASE 6.5: GROOVED TONGUE

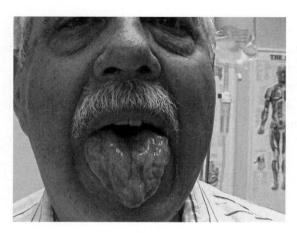

VIDEO 6.5

A 45-year-old diabetic man presented with a 5-year history of intermittent diplopia and feet numbness. Examination is shown. He also had mild sensory impairment in the feet and absent ankle jerks. Nerve conduction study revealed mild sensory neuropathy.

The following tongue abnormalities are not uncommonly seen in chronic MG:

1. Weakness
2. Atrophy
3. Grooving
4. Fasciculations
5. All of the above

DIAGNOSIS

- The video showed mild fatigable right ptosis and grooved tongue.
- In chronic MG, atrophy of the tongue leads to formation of triple furrowed appearance with grooves paralleling median sulcus in each side.
- Tongue atrophy and weakness are commonly seen in MuSK MG.
- Tongue fasciculations are not a feature of MG (there is one questionable case report in the medical literature).

CASE 6.6: FAMILIAL MUSCLE STIFFNESS

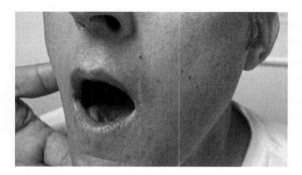

VIDEO 6.6

A 38-year-old man had developed symptoms since age 21 years that consisted of muscle stiffness, painful muscle spasms, difficulty chewing, and memory problems. He had several cousins and a sister with the same symptoms. His tongue examination is shown.

This demonstrated reaction of the tongue is due to:

1. Atrophy
2. Myotonia
3. Pain
4. Weakness
5. Reaction to the cotton in the Q-tip

DIAGNOSIS

- The video showed persistent grooving of the tongue after applying pressure with a Q-tip.
- In patients with a myotonic disorder, myotonia can be:
  - Spontaneous, affecting extremities during walking or running leading to falls
  - Induced by:
    - Percussion of selected muscles such as
      - Thenar eminence: percussion leads to sustained abduction or opposition of the thumb.
      - Wrist extensors: percussion leads to sustained wrist extension.
    - Pressure: application of sustained pressure on the tongue, leads to grooving due to sustained poor relaxation of the pressed muscles. Percussion of the tongue may produce the same, but it is more technically difficult to perform.
    - Gripping: grip myotonia leads to difficulty in relaxation of finger flexors after a forceful handshake.
- It is important when examining for myotonia to repeat the tapping or pressure in order to examine for "warming up" phenomenon, which means improvement of relaxation of the affected muscle by repeated challenge. This is typically seen in myotonia. On the other hand, paramyotonia (PMC) worsens with repeated challenge. Cold has the same effect on PMC.
- Myotonia of the tongue explains dysarthria in these patients and cold-induced dysarthria in patients with sodium channelopathies.
- Tongue myotonia is more pronounced than grip myotonia in myotonic dystrophy type 2.
- In our experience, tongue myotonia responds to Mexiletine as well as grip myotonia.

CASE 6.7: TONGUE TWITCHING AFTER RADIOTHERAPY

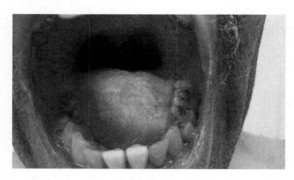

VIDEO 6.7

A 53-year-old male presented with trouble swallowing and excessive drooling. His examination is shown. Deep tendon reflexes were revealed as normal. Clinical findings did not change when he was seen 5 years later.

Tongue fasciculation occurs in all the following conditions except:

1. Amyotrophic lateral sclerosis
2. Kennedy disease
3. After radiotherapy
4. Organophosphorous compounds poisoning
5. Snake venom poisoning

DIAGNOSIS

- The video showed dysarthria, tongue fasciculations, excessive salivation, and atrophy of the cervical muscles.
- Effect of radiation on the nervous system can be:
  - Acute
  - Subacute
  - Remote
- Remote effect of radiation may appear several years later in the form of motor neuron dysfunction in the irradiated area.
- Painless atrophy, weakness, and fasciculation may lead to diagnostic confusion with ALS.
  - Unlike ALS, DTRs are usually absent in the affected area and the course is not relentless.
- A typical course is that of initial worsening then stabilization.
- Myokymia in EMG is a highly characteristic sign.
- While ALS is the most ominous cause of tongue fasciculations, other causes should be born in mind, which include:
  - Lower motor neuron disease (Kennedy disease, spinal muscular atrophy, poliomyelitis)
  - Brainstem lesions
  - Base of skull tumor
  - Skull base irradiation
  - Hypoglossal neuropathy
  - Organophosphorus poisoning
  - Snake venom poisoning
- Tongue weakness is an important sign and can precede fasciculations and atrophy in lower motor neuron syndromes and neuromuscular junction disorders. Strength of the tongue muscles is tested by asking the patient to push the tongue against the check and against the examiner's finger from outside.
- Advanced ALS patients may be unable to move their tongues at all. They are usually anarthritic.
- Irradiation of para-aortic lymph nodes for lymphoma or testicular tumors may produce LMN syndrome in the legs years later.
- It is always important to ask about history of irradiation in patients with fasciculations and atrophy because patients do not think of such connections and may not volunteer such information.

CASE 6.8: UNEXPECTED EMG FINDING

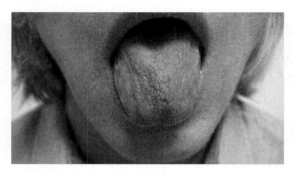

VIDEO 6.8

A 61-year-old woman presented with bilateral hand pain that prompted an EMG, which revealed widespread spontaneous activity and tongue movements as shown in the video. She was referred for confirmation of "ALS." Her examination revealed percussion myotonia of the thenar muscles that worsened with repeated tapping (paramyotonia), and the EMG showed diffuse myotonic discharges. She had abnormal sodium channel (SCNA) mutation consistent with paramyotonia congenita that was asymptomatic. The tongue had normal bulk and strength and showed rhythmic contractions that were part of her essential tremor.

Unlike tremor of the tongue, ALS-related fasciculations are:

1. Irregular
2. Frequent
3. Associated with weakness and atrophy
4. 1, 2, and 3
5. 1 and 3

DIAGNOSIS

- Tongue tremor is a common finding and is usually part of essential or physiological tremor.
- It is regular and has a frequency of 6–10 HZ.
- Sometimes, tongue tremor is punctuated by "jerks," leading to even more confusion with fasciculations.
- The tongue is not weak and not atrophied. It is important to inspect and examine the strength of the tongue in all cases of abnormal tongue movement to look for atrophy and weakness.
- Normal jaw jerk supports the benign nature of the abnormal tongue movement.
- Needle EMG of the extrinsic tongue muscles revealed rhythmic contractions and motor units with normal configuration and firing frequency.
- Fasciculations of ALS are irregular, infrequent, and associated with atrophy and weakness of the tongue.

CASE 6.9: FACIAL TWITCHING AND LARGE BREASTS

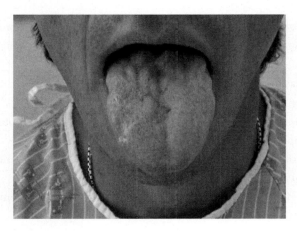

VIDEO 6.9

A 42-year-old man from Mexico had noticed facial twitching whenever he became nervous since age 20 years. A few years later he noticed mild slurring of speech. His examination is shown. Genetic testing was diagnostic.

Mutation of which gene is expected in this case?

1. Androgen receptors (AR)
2. Superoxide dismutase (SOD)
3. Valosin containing protein
4. TAR DNA-binding protein 43 (TDP-43)
5. Fused in Sarcoma (FUS)

DIAGNOSIS

- The video showed atrophy and fasciculations of the tongue, abnormal facial movements, and large breasts (gynecomastia). These findings are very suggestive of Kennedy disease.
- Kennedy disease is an X-linked spinal muscular atrophy.
- Mean age of onset of symptoms is 27 years.
- Due to mutation of androgen receptors, affected males display impotence, gynecomastia, testicular atrophy, and infertility.
- The presence of muscle cramps, proximal symmetrical weakness, and elevated CK leads to suspicion of a myopathy.
- The presence of feet numbness and areflexia leads to suspicion of neuropathy. Nerve conduction study (NCS) usually shows mild sensory neuropathy.
- Dysphagia, dysarthria, and fatigability of chewing muscles and dropped jaw (due to trigeminal palsy) leads to suspicion of MG.
- Any young male with proximal weakness and neurogenic EMG should be examined for Kennedy disease.
- Molecular basis: CAG repeat expansion (40–65 repeats). Androgen plays a role in cell survival and dendritic growth.
- A heterozygous female may show tongue fasciculations and muscle cramps in the 7th decade.
- An autosomal dominant clinical variant of Kennedy disease is reported with no clear identification of the molecular basis yet.

CASE 6.10: RESTLESS TONGUE

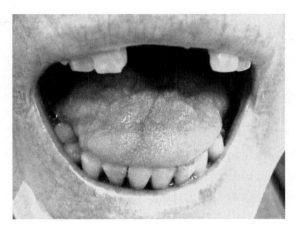

VIDEO 6.10

A 76-year-old man who had radiotherapy for carcinoma of the tonsils 20 years earlier presented with dysphagia and excessive drooling. Examination showed atrophy and spontaneous movements of the tongue and absent jaw jerk. EMG of the tongue revealed bursts of discharges at a semi-rhythmic pattern.

The shown activity is reported in all the following conditions except:

1. Delayed post-irradiation motor neuron disease (MND)
2. Bell palsy
3. Episodic ataxia 1
4. Radiation-induced plexopathy
5. Myopathy

DIAGNOSIS

The video showed atrophy and myokymia of the tongue, which is confirmed by EMG.

Myokymia:

- Single MUAP firing as bursts of multiplet
- 30–40 Hz discharges in short bursts
- Burst occur at 2–10 Hz
- Burst duration is 100–900 msc
- Semi-rhythmic burst pattern
- Bursts start and stop abruptly
- Spontaneous

Causes of myokymia:

- Brainstem glioma
- Multiple sclerosis (MS)
- Neuromyotonia
- Benign fasciculation syndrome
- Traumatic and inflammatory neuropathies such as Bell palsy
- Post-irradiation neuronopathy
- Episodic ataxia

Delayed post-irradiation toxicity to motor neurons is well recognized and usually occurs years after exposure. Myokymia is very characteristic.

CASE 6.11: NECK PAIN AND TONGUE DEVIATION

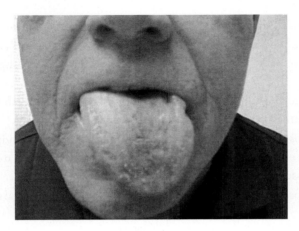

VIDEO 6.11

A 56-year-old man presented with acute left neck pain followed by dysarthria. A few months later the shown examination was made.

The most likely cause for these findings is:

1. Brainstem tumor
2. Trauma to the tongue
3. Carotid artery dissection
4. Jugular foramen tumor
5. Stroke

DIAGNOSIS

- The video showed left tongue deviation.
- The hypoglossal nerves are the motor nerves to the tongue, and can be affected anywhere in their pathway from their origin in the medulla oblongata to the tongue muscles.
- Unilateral hypoglossal palsy leads to deviation of the tongue to the weak side (unlike paralyzed palate where the uvula deviates to the healthy side).
- Important causes of hypoglossal palsy from the neuromuscular standpoint include:
  - Hereditary neuropathy with liability to pressure palsy (HNPP): usually there is a history of pressure such as sleeping with jaw supported by an arm leading to pressure on the hypoglossal nerve. There is a history of other self-limiting focal neuropathies in the past.
  - Carotid artery dissection: usually caused by trauma to the neck. Common findings are acute neck pain and Horner syndrome due to interruption of the sympathetic fibers to the ipsilateral pupil, which are conveyed via carotid arteries. This is the right answer.
  - As a part of Parsonage Turner syndrome (hypoglossal nerves are less commonly affected than anterior interosseus, suprascapular, long thoracic, and phrenic nerves).
  - Glomus tumor: usually hypoglossal nerve is affected along with other lower cranial nerves. Progression is usually slow.
  - Idiopathic (usually acute and self-limiting, similar to Bell palsy).
- Patients with more diffuse diseases like ALS and Kennedy disease may present with slight tongue asymmetry resulting from tongue atrophy, but unilateral tongue weakness is not a feature.

CASE 6.12: MUSCLE STIFFNESS AND WINTER WEAKNESS

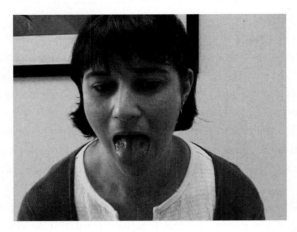

VIDEO 6.12

A 40-year-old woman developed painful muscle stiffness, especially during winters, and episodic generalized weakness, usually after heavy meals. There was no family history of significance. Examination of the tongue is shown. She had a positive genetic testing.

The expected mutation affects the gene of the following:

1. Sodium channel
2. Calcium channel
3. Potassium channel
4. Chloride channel
5. None of the above

DIAGNOSIS

- The video showed percussion myotonia of the tongue. Her EMG revealed generalized myotonic discharges.
- Myotonia is characterized by the persistence of strong contraction of muscle after stimulation has ceased. The contraction can be initiated voluntarily, mechanically, or electrically.
- Percussion of the tongue leads to localized constriction (napkin ring sign).
- Tongue myotonia is not specific to any myotonic disorder.
- Worsening of myotonia with repeated testing and cold suggests sodium channelopathy.
- Periodic weakness suggests hyperkalemic periodic paralysis, which is allelic to paramyotonia congenita (PMC). It usually starts in adolescence and each episode lasts less than 2 hours.
- PMC is caused by a sodium channel (SCN4A) mutation.
- Prolonged decrease of compound muscle action potential (CMAP) amplitude with long exercise test is typical.
- Mexiletine 150 mg–1,000 mg a day is effective by blocking sodium channels.
- Hyperkalemic periodic paralysis usually responds to hydrochlorothiazide or acetazolamide therapy.

CASE 6.13: EAR PAIN AND TONGUE DEVIATION

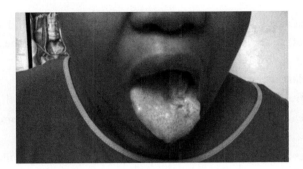

VIDEO 6.13

A 41-year-old woman presented with a 1-year history of tinnitus and left otalgia, followed by the mentioned symptoms and demonstrated signs.

The most likely cause of the left tongue atrophy in this case is:

1. Carotid dissection
2. Parsonage Turner syndrome
3. Cavernous sinus pathology
4. Retro-orbital pathology
5. Glomus jugulare

DIAGNOSIS

- Hearing impairment, vocal cord paralysis, tongue deviation, and facial pain suggest involvement of the 8th, 10th, 12th, and 5th cranial nerves. Among the mentioned choices, glomus jugulare is the only one that can be that extensive.
- Glomus Jugulare is a neuroendocrine neoplasm. 97% are benign.
- It originates from paraganglia in chromaffin negative glomus cells that are derived from embryonic neural crest. Seventy-five percent are sporadic, asymptomatic, or cause painless masses.
- Common sites are head and neck, and mostly it originates in the middle ear and spreads to the jugular foramen and beyond, leading to multiple compressive cranial neuropathies.
- It is a slowly evolving tumor that appears at age 40–70 years.
- Symptoms usually start with tinnitus, conductive hearing loss, and as it progresses it leads to vertigo, nystagmus, and facial palsy.
- Jugular foramen pathology symptoms:
  - 9th and 10th: dysphonia, dysphagia
  - 11th: weak trapezius and sternocleidomastoid muscle
  - 12th: tongue hemiatrophy
- Carotid canal: Horner syndrome
- 5th and 6th cranial nerves symptoms indicate inoperability.
- Radiation surgery usually leads to a cure or long-term control.
- Carotid dissection may lead to hypoglossal palsy but does not extend to the abducens or trigeminal nerve.
- Cavernous sinus pathology may lead to involvement of the 3rd–5th cranial nerves but does not extend to the hypoglossal nerve.
- Retrorbital pathology does not go that far either.
- Parsonage Turner may cause hypoglossal neuropathy but does not affect the rest of the cranial nerves.

DYSARTHRIA

CASE 7.1: CRYING AND LAUGHTER

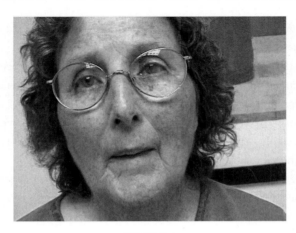

VIDEO 7.1

A 63-year-old woman presented with a 6-month history of speech difficulty and outbursts of laughter and crying that were not provoked and sometimes socially inappropriate. Three months later, she developed swallowing difficulty. Her examination revealed tongue atrophy and fasciculations and brisk jaw jerk.

Statements below regarding dysarthria in amyotrophic lateral sclerosis (ALS) are true except:

1. It usually precedes dysphagia.
2. It usually follows dysphagia.
3. It is associated with tongue weakness.
4. It is usually of mixed upper motor neuron (UMN) and lower motor neuron (LMN) type.
5. It is associated with poor prognosis.

DIAGNOSIS

- Dysarthria in ALS occurs in 80% of cases. Only in 25% of cases, dysarthria is the first symptom of the disease.
- It is estimated that dysarthria appears after 80% of motor neurons are lost.
- The average time between the onset of dysarthria and the diagnosis of ALS ranges from 33 months before the diagnosis to 60 months after the diagnosis.
- As an initial symptom, dysarthria is eight times more common than dysphagia.
- ALS patients usually have mixed flaccid and spastic dysarthria, but there is no cerebellar element in it; therefore, it is regular.
  - In some cases, flaccid dysarthria predominates (weakness is proportional to atrophy).
  - In other cases, spastic dysarthria is the only presenting symptom, posing a diagnostic challenge. No atrophy or fasciculations of the tongue are noticed and the jaw jerk is brisk. Side to side tongue movement is slow.
- Speech in ALS is characterized by being slow, laborious, imprecise consonant production, hypernasality, emission of air during speech, and hoarseness.
- Other bulbar symptoms like emotional lability and dyspnea coexist.
- Dysarthria eventually progress to anarthria, imposing serious communication problems and social isolation. Therefore, it is important to adopt new communication strategies before anarthria occurs.
- Tongue weakness is an important cause of dysarthria in ALS patients and it is an independent risk factor for poor survival.
- Speech disturbances in ALS may also be related to concomitant frontotemporal dementia, dysphonia, or breathing problems.

REFERENCE

Tomik B, et al. Dysarthria in ALS: a review. *ALS*. 2010;11:4–15.

CASE 7.2: DYSARTHRIA AND FALLS

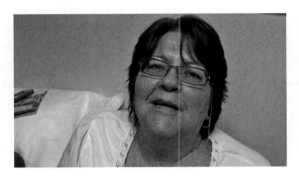

VIDEO 7.2

A 57-year-old woman was referred for a 2-year history of progressive loss of balance, speech difficulty, and hyperreflexia. Magnetic resonance imaging (MRI) of the brain and spinal cord revealed nonspecific white matter lesions in the brainstem and cerebellum. Cerebrospinal fluid (CSF) was positive for oligoclonal bands.

Unlike that of ALS, dysarthria of progressive multiple sclerosis (MS) is usually associated with:

1. Jaw hyperreflexia
2. Tongue atrophy
3. Irregular rhythm
4. Dyspnea
5. Emotional lability

DIAGNOSIS

- Examination showed scanning speech and dysdiadochokinesia.
- Patients with progressive dysarthria are referred for neuromuscular evaluation due to suspicion of ALS or myasthenia gravis (MG). However, many of them end up having a non-neuromuscular diagnosis such as MS, cerebrovascular disease, movement disorders, or functional etiology. Therefore, a neuromuscular specialist needs to learn about these diseases and the pattern of speech disturbances in them.

Dysarthria in MS is:

- Usually of mixed type: spastic and cerebellar due to vulnerability of the cerebellum and corticobulbar tracts to MS pathology. No lower motor neuron (LMN) signs are expected, such as tongue atrophy or fasciculations.
- Cerebellar elements are suggested by the irregularity of dysarthria and the presence of ataxia, dysmetria, nystagmus, and dysdiadochokinesia.
- It is slowly progressive or relapsing-remitting, depending on the type of MS. In relapsing-remitting MS (RRMS), acute dysarthria and ataxia may be misdiagnosed as a stroke, while in progressive MS, dysarthria may be misdiagnosed as ALS.
- The cerebellar element (if present) facilitates the diagnosis, but difficulty arises when the dysarthria is spastic and progressive. Of course, one will have to find evidence of demyelination in other sites and/or times.
- Emotional lability usually exists and it is different than that of ALS by being more of decreased crying or laughter threshold than classic paroxysmal giggling.

REFERENCE

Hartelius L, Runmarker B, Andersen O. Prevalence and characteristics of dysarthria in a multiple-sclerosis incidence cohort: relation to neurological data. *Folia Phoniatr Logop.* 2000 Jul–Aug;52(4):160–177.

CASE 7.3: RELAPSING REMITTING DYSARTHRIA

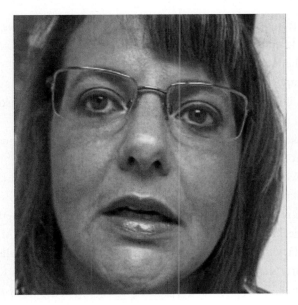

VIDEO 7.3

A 33-year-old woman presented with acute dysarthria and ataxia that responded to steroids. She had multiple white matter lesions in the brainstem and cerebellum and positive oligoclonal bands (OCBs) in the CSF. She had multiple relapses in the following few years.

The most likely diagnosis is:

1. Amyotrophic lateral sclerosis (ALS)
2. Myasthenia gravis (MG)
3. Multiple sclerosis (MS)
4. Chronic inflammatory demyelinating polyneuropathy (CIDP)
5. Neuromyelitis optica (NMO)

DIAGNOSIS

- This case illustrates similar findings to case 7.2, but the symptoms were intermittent.
- Examination demonstrated explosive irregular speech, cerebellar ataxia, impaired heel to shin test, dysdiadochokinesia, and hyperreflexia.
- Dysarthria simply means difficulty with articulation.
- Anatomically, it is either flaccid (LMN disorder), spastic (UMN disorder), or cerebellar (irregular).
- In ALS, it is usually of mixed UMN and LMN type. Cerebellar quality should raise a question about the diagnosis of ALS.
- In MS, it is usually of mixed spastic and cerebellar type; any LMN findings should raise a question about the diagnosis.
- Multisystem atrophy may also produce spastic/cerebellar type dysarthria. The age group tends to be older, and no evidence of demyelination is found on the MRIs.
- Cerebrovascular disease may also produce mixed spastic and cerebellar dysarthria.
- LMN dysarthria may be caused by other forms of MND such as Kennedy disease or post-irradiation bulbar palsy. Other clinical pictures and the time course are important to differentiate.
- MG is the most challenging differential diagnosis, especially MuSK Ab associated MG, which tends to affect bulbar muscles more than the ocular muscles. MuSK MG may cause atrophy of the pharyngeal, tongue, or facial muscles, and there are case reports of tongue fasciculations.
- Repetitive nerve stimulation test is abnormal in 25% of ALS cases, and negative MG serology in seen in 20% of MG cases.
- Mild worsening of symptoms in the evenings is common in ALS.
- Positive single fiber electromyogram (SFEMG) is common in ALS.
- From what has been said, the diagnosis of bulbar ALS or MG may be delayed until other findings appear to make the diagnosis clearer.
- A therapeutic trial of prednisone may help the diagnosis. A negative 6-week trial of prednisone 1 mg/kg of body weight would strongly argue against MG. Initial worsening of symptoms of MG after initiation of steroids should not be held against the diagnosis of MG as 7%–15% of cases worsen within 2 weeks of initiation. Myasthenic crisis can be induced with steroids, in particular in those with bulbar dysfunction.

CASE 7.4: SPASTIC DYSARTHRIA

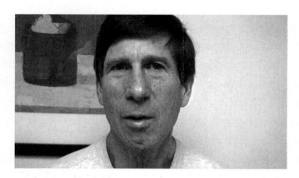

VIDEO 7.4

A 62-year-old man presented with a 1-year history of speech difficulty. His tongue was not atrophied and did not show fasciculations but it was weak and the jaw jerk was brisk. There was no major dysphagia or diplopia and there was no weakness of the extremities. The electromyogram (EMG) was normal, including the tongue. Brain MRI was normal. Gradually he became more dysarthric and more spastic in the legs. AChR antibody titer was 0.9 nmol/L.

The most likely diagnosis is:

1. Bulbar MG
2. MuSK MG
3. Bulbar onset primary lateral sclerosis (PLS)
4. Bulbar onset ALS
5. Brainstem tumor

DIAGNOSIS

- The examination showed spastic dysarthria and hyperreflexia.
- A variant of ALS in which degeneration is restricted to the upper motor neurons has been recognized for many years and is called primary lateral sclerosis (PLS).
- It usually affects males around age 50 years, starting in the legs in 87% of cases, which leads to spastic gait.
- Eventually, pseudobulbar symptoms occur in 40% of cases, but rarely are they the presenting features. Asymmetry is noticed in 50% of cases.
- Lower extremity onset cases are confused with myelopathies. Neuroimaging excludes compressive etiology but non-compressive myelopathies can be challenging to sort out. These may include B_{12} and copper deficiency, hereditary spastic paraplegia, MS, and adrenomyeloneuropathy.
- Bulbar onset PLS remains a diagnosis of exclusion.
- The following tests are usually performed to rule out other causes: MG serology, EMG, brain MRI, CSF examination, hereditary spastic paraplegia mutation analysis, B_{12} and copper levels.
- A weakly positive AChR antibody titer is reported in ALS and should not lead to erroneous diagnosis of MG and subsequent unnecessary immunosupression. MG does not cause spastic dysarthria.
- The course of PLS is progressive and in some cases progresses to a full-blown ALS.

CASE 7.5: DYSARTHRIA LONG AFTER RADIOTHERAPY

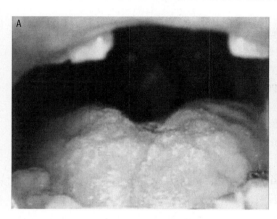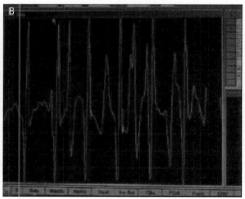

VIDEO 7.5

A 76-year-old man presented with a 2-year history of slurring of speech and swallowing difficulty. Past medical history was remarkable for cancer of the tonsils treated with radiation 20 years earlier. Examination and EMG of the tongue are shown in Video 7.5A and 7.5B, respectively. He worsened for a year and needed a percutaneous endoscopic gastrostomy (PEG) tube placement, then stabilized. This video was taken 10 years later.

The demonstrated EMG discharges are:

1. Fasciculations
2. Complex repetitive discharges
3. Myokymia
4. Myotonic discharges
5. Voluntary activity

The following is correct regarding post-irradiation bulbar palsy:

1. It may occur years after exposure to radiation.
2. It follows the same course as ALS.
3. Myokymia is a typical EMG feature.
4. It does not occur with low dose irradiation.
5. Usually, it resolves spontaneously.

DIAGNOSIS

- The video shows myokymia of the tongue and restriction of movement of the soft palate.
- It occurs in 10% of patients treated with radiation directed to the neck region. It can happen even with exposure to a small dose of radiation.
- Bulbar palsy is often accompanied by cervical amyotrophy, hypoglossal nerve palsy, and Horner syndrome.
- Average time of onset after exposure is 5.5 years.
- Symptoms may progress for years before they reach a plateau. Spontaneous resolution does not occur.
- The subacute onset and subsequent stuttering of symptoms support vascular etiology rather than a direct neuronal toxicity.
- A similar picture of motor neuron disease may evolve in the lumbar region after irradiation of the pelvic area.
- Chronic denervation in the affected areas and sometimes beyond is reported. More specifically, myokymia is seen in the vast majority of cases.

REFERENCE

Chew NK, et al. Delayed post-irradiation bulbar palsy in nasopharyngeal carcinoma. *Neurology.* 2001 Aug 14; 57(3):529–531.

CASE 7.6: FAMILIAL DYSARTHRIA, SENSORY ATAXIA, AND ELEVATED CK

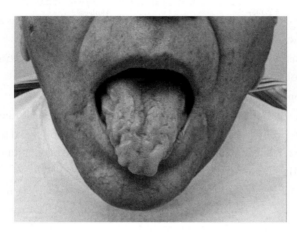

VIDEO 7.6

An 80-year-old man presented with a 10-year history of slurring of speech, weakness and atrophy of the legs and arms, and loss of balance. Examination revealed sensory ataxia, impaired feet sensation to vibration, diffuse areflexia, fasciculations of the face and chest muscles, and weakness of the tongue and face. Speech was nasal. EMG revealed widespread chronic denervation of the legs, arms, and tongue. CPK level was 1,500 U/L. He had a brother with similar symptoms.

Which of the following is the most likely diagnosis:

1. Chronic myopathy
2. Axonal neuropathy
3. Kennedy disease
4. Acid maltase deficiency
5. ALS

DIAGNOSIS

- The video showed gynecomastia and nasal speech. Due to the presence of chronic diffuse denervation, bulbar symptoms, and gynecomastia, mutation analysis for androgen receptor mutations was obtained and it was positive.
- Kennedy disease is an X-linked recessive disease caused by mutation of the androgen receptor gene on Xq12.
    - The mutation is in the form of CAG repeat expansion.
    - Most affected people have a repeat number of 40–65 (normal range is 10–36).
    - CTG repeats produce polyglutamate tail, which leads to abnormal folding of the androgen receptors, resulting in partial proteolysis. Androgen plays a role in cell survival and dendritic growth.
    - Autosomal dominant bulbospinal atrophy with gynecomastia is also reported.
- Pathologically, the disease is characterized by degeneration of the motor and sensory neurons. Extraocular muscles are spared.
- Age of onset: 15–60 years.
- Heterozygous females may display tongue fasciculations and muscle cramps in the 7th decade.
- Muscle cramps, fatigue, and leg weakness are common early symptoms.
- Full-blown picture:
    - Proximal weakness, atrophy, and fasciculations.
    - Tongue weakness and fasciculations.
    - Facial myokymia
    - Dysphagia, dysarthria
    - Diffuse areflexia
    - Reduced sensation in the feet and hands and small sensory nerve action potentials (SNAPS)
    - Action tremor
    - Gynecomastia, testicular atrophy, erectile dysfunction
    - Diabetes mellitus
- Needle electromyography: chronic diffuse denervation expressed as giant motor units potentials with fast firing rate.
- Mildly elevated creatine kinase (CK).
- It affects 2:100,000 of population.
- Every male with muscle cramps, high CK, and neurogenic EMG should be tested for Kennedy disease, especially if there is gynecomastia or bulbar weakness.
- In chronic motor neuron disorders, the presence of high CK and low sensory nerve action potentials (SNAPS) should raise the possibility of Kennedy disease.

CASE 7.7: CEREBELLAR ATAXIA AND TONGUE FASCICULATIONS

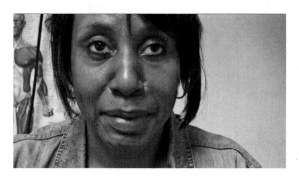

VIDEO 7.7

A 43-year-old woman presented with a 10-year history of twitching of the facial muscles and loss of balance. Brain MRI revealed mild cerebellar atrophy. EMG confirmed fasciculations of the face and tongue but there was no widespread denervation.

The most likely diagnosis is:

1. Spinocerebellar ataxia (SCA) type 3
2. Kennedy disease
3. SCA type 2
4. Familial ALS
5. Friedreich ataxia

DIAGNOSIS

- Weakness of the tongue is a feature of:
  - Bulbar and pseudobulbar palsy: ALS, Kennedy disease, and other motor neuron disorders. The weakness is associated with atrophy and fasciculations except in PLS cases.
  - Neuromuscular junction disorders like MG. Atrophy is not a feature except in MuSK MG. Fluctuation of symptoms is typical.
  - Hypoglossal palsy: brainstem pathology, hypoglossal neuropathy such as neuritis or carotid dissection, and so on. This is usually unilateral and is associated with atrophy.
- Dysarthria is a product of interference with articulation mechanism and it could be:
  - Labial
  - Lingual
  - Palatal
  - Facial: Bell palsy
- Lingual dysarthria is characterized by difficulty pronouncing lingual sounds like T, L, and D.
- In ALS, tongue weakness is almost always present by the time dysarthria appears. It is important to examine tongue strength by asking the patient to push the tongue against the cheek and the examiner's finger from outside.
- In MG, the weakness is intermittent and gets worse with repetition. Tongue weakness may not be appreciated by examination.
- Labial dysarthria usually accompanies lingual dysarthria in MG.
- What makes the diagnosis more difficult is that myasthenia serology and repetitive nerve stimulation (RNS) test is negative in 40% of bulbar MG cases.
- Functional weakness is difficult to exclude, and many cases of MG are considered to be hysterical initially. Precipitation and relief of symptoms in relation to stress is not uncommon in MG.
- Negative response to steroids is seen in only 10% of MG cases and therefore argues the most against the diagnosis of MG.
- Negative SFEMG of a weak muscle argues strongly against MG.
- The speech of this lady returned to normal few months after her divorce and new marriage to her new boyfriend.

CASE 7.9: NASAL SPEECH AND HYPERCKEMIA

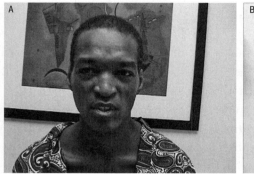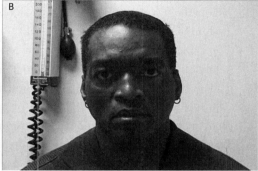

VIDEO 7.9

A 36-year-old man presented with a 4-week history of progressive nasal speech, dysphagia, and proximal and distal weakness of the extremities. He lost 30 pounds. EMG showed the demonstrated activity in the arms, legs, and thoracic paraspinal muscles. Nerve conduction study (NCS) was normal. CPK level was 2210 U/L. Erythrocyte sedimentation rate (ESR) was 74 mm/hour. He did not respond to 60 mg/day of prednisone given for 6 weeks. Muscle pathology is shown (Figure 7.9.1). There was also severe endomysial inflammation that consisted mainly of CD4 cells.

These pathological findings are typically seen in:

1. Dermatomyositis
2. ALS
3. Spinal muscular atrophy (SMA)
4. Polymyositis
5. Inclusion body myositis (IBM)

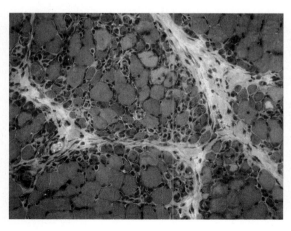

FIGURE 7.9.1 H &E stain, 100x.

DIAGNOSIS

- The pathology picture shows perifascicular atrophy (atrophy of multiple layers on the margin of the fascicles due to ischemia).
- The typical presentation of dermatomyositis is that of subacute symmetrical proximal weakness, periorbital swelling, violaceous rash on the knuckles, Gottron sign, elevated CK, and irritative myopathy in EMG and normal sensory system. Reflexes are usually normal.
- The typical ALS presentation is that of progressive dysarthria, dysphagia, distal more than proximal weakness and atrophy, hyperreflexia, and normal sensory system. CK may be mildly elevated and EMG shows widespread denervation.
- In this case, an alternative diagnosis to ALS was sought due to the following factors:
  - The lack of atrophy despite severe weakness.
  - Weight loss in ALS occurs late and is proportional to dysphagia and low intake.
  - Dysphonia and nasal speech are not common in ALS. Instead, rather dysarthria is typically seen and it precedes dysphagia.
  - Elevated CK: while hyperCKemia is common in denervated conditions like ALS, the CK level is usually below 1,000 U/L.
  - Elevated ESR, although not specific, along with weight loss, suggested systemic inflammation.
  - Bilateral foot drop with preservation of the bulk of extensor digitorum brevis (EBD). In ALS, EDB mass is lost due to neurogenic atrophy.
  - Due to these factors, a muscle biopsy was done and it revealed:
    - Endomysial and perivascular mononuclear inflammatory cells infiltration
    - Predominance of CD4 in the inflammatory infiltrate
    - Perifascicular atrophy as shown in Figure 7.9.1
    - Positive MAC antibody reaction
- Nasal speech is not common in dermatomyositis, and we speculate that inflammation and weakness of the palatine muscles is responsible for this finding.
- Skin rash is not required for the diagnosis of dermatomyositis. Pathological findings are specific and can differentiate it from other inflammatory muscle diseases.
- The patient returned to normal strength after treatment with IV cyclophosphamide (Video 7.9B).

CASE 7.10: THYMECTOMY OR NOT?

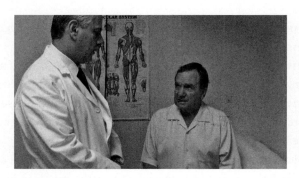

VIDEO 7.10

A 69-year-old man presented with a 2-month history of speech difficulty. AChR antibody titer was 23 nmol/l. He had a history of a large ascending aortic aneurysm, coronary artery disease, and prostate cancer.

(True/false) Thymectomy in this case is advisable.

DIAGNOSIS

- The video examination revealed labial and lingual dysarthria with a nasal component, facial weakness, and fatigability of the proximal leg muscles.
- Thymectomy is indicated for thymoma, which occurs in 5%–15% of myasthenics.
- For non-thymomatous myasthenics, thymectomy is generally advised for all patients with generalized MG of age 10–65 years. In our practice we advise it up to 70 years if the patients are healthy otherwise. This patient has many comorbid conditions beside his borderline age limit; therefore we did not advise it.
- There is no role for emergency thymectomy since its impact will not appear before a year.
- The thymus gland plays an important role in the pathogenesis of MG mostly due to the presence of "myoid cells" in the thymus that have molecular similarities with the nicotinic post-synaptic ACh receptors.
- Retrospective studies have shown increased long-term remission rate of MG after thymectomy compared to non-thymectomized patients.
- The practice of thymectomy has been performed for more than 50 years since Blalock published a series of poorly controlled non-thymomatous myasthenics who improved dramatically after thymectomy.
- Thymic hyperplasia is seen in the majority of these patients pathologically.
- In the elderly, the thymus is reduced to a small tag that is difficult to identify and it is not pathologically active anyway. Therefore, thymectomy is not indicated.
- Transternal thymectomy is more likely to remove any ectopic thymic tissue. It is preferred in patients with thymoma. Transcervical thymectomy has become popular and may be as effective.
- Interestingly, MuSK antibodies associated MG may not be as responsive to thymectomy, and therefore surgery is not indicated.
- A recently completed multicenter double blind trial on the impact of thymectomy on treatment of MG in non-thymomatous patients will hopefully provide some evidence-based answers to the question of thymectomy in MG.

CASE 7.11: MORBIDITY IN ALS: CAN IT BE IMPROVED?

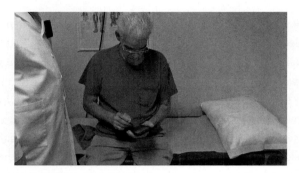

VIDEO 7.11

A 70-year-old man presented with a 6-month history of progressive speech difficulty, cough, orthopnea, weight loss, and excessive salivation. Examination revealed (in addition to what is shown in the video) atrophy and fasciculations of the tongue, diffuse hyperreflexia, and normal cognition and strength of the extremities. Myasthenia serology was negative. Sensory and motor nerve conduction studies were normal. Needle examination of the extremities and thoracic paraspinal muscles was normal, but the tongue was denervated. CPK level was 450 U/L. Bain MRI was normal.

Which of the following can improve quality of life in bulbar ALS:

1. PEG tube
2. Biphasic positive airway pressure (BIPAP)
3. Botulinum toxin for refractory hypersialosis
4. Electronic communication system
5. All of the above

DIAGNOSIS

- Bulbar involvement is a bad prognostic sign in ALS. Serial assessment of bulbar functions is recommended in these patients.
- There are certain measures that are shown to reduce morbidity and improve lifestyle in ALS patients with bulbar dysfunction.
  1. Dysphagia: early PEG placement is important to reduce more loss of muscle mass, which may worsen respiratory insufficiency due to its effect on the respiratory muscles. Cough, voice change, and weight loss are early signs of aspiration. Recurrent pneumonia is a late sign. Modified barium swallow may cause aspiration. The isosmolar contrast agent Iotrolan, which has no significant adverse effects even in the case of aspiration, is recommended.
  2. Dyspnea: early institution of BiPAP helps sleep apnea and improves sleep and, secondarily, reduces daytime fatigue and lack of concentration.
  3. Dysarthria: early institution of a communication system is important to reduce incidence of depression and poor healthcare delivery due to lack of communication. Electronic communication devices with a keyboard or a scanner to detect head or eye movements and with a voice output enable patients to use telephones and computers in a very effective way. Patients can be sent for recording of their voice patterns before they develop severe dysarthria so that the communicative device can be programmed with their own voice instead of a robotic sound.
  4. Sialorrhea: anticholinergic drugs, like nortriptyline 25–75 mg at bedtime or glycopyrrolate 1–2 mg daily, are usually effective. Refractory cases may benefit from botulinum toxin injection to the salivary glands. Surprisingly, worsening of dysphagia is not encountered as much as expected.
  5. Emotional lability: this is due to involvement of the suprabulbar pathways and may not be associated with depression. Tricyclic antidepressant drugs like nortriptyline usually help. Nuedexta (dextromethorphan/quinidine) is also shown to be effective.

REFERENCE

Kühnlein P, et al. Diagnosis and treatment of bulbar symptoms in amyotrophic lateral sclerosis. *Nature Clinical Practice Neurology*. 2008;4:366–374.

CASE 7.12A: SELF-MEDICATED MYASTHENIC

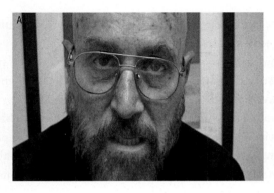

VIDEO 7.12A

A 56-year-old man presented with nasal speech and diplopia. AChR antibody titer was 24 nmol/L. He responded well to prednisone, but after 3 months he discontinued it and started taking short courses only when his symptoms exacerbated.

Poor compliance in MG is probably:

1. More common than in CIDP
2. More common in young female patients
3. Contributes to poor outcome
4. PRN steroid administration by patients is as effective as chronic steroid administration by a neurologist
5. Overall side effects of PRN steroids in MG are less than chronic use

DIAGNOSIS

- Poor treatment compliance (PTC) in MG accounts for 23% of unsatisfactory outcome rates, which are estimated to be 20%.
- The phenomenon of poor compliance in MG has not been studied systematically in terms of its characteristics, impact, and solutions; therefore, the following discussion is based on our experience.
- The most common causes and risk factors of poor compliance in MG are:
  - Side effects of steroids that can be disabling and disfiguring, in particular weight gain.
  - Poor treatment compliance is more common in females, especially young females.
  - The fluctuating nature of the disease enforces the feeling by some patients that they do not need to be treated continuously.
  - The good response of the symptoms to treatment with reversal to normal function tempts some patients to change the dosage or to quit medications on their own.
- Poor compliance may take the following forms:
  - Discontinuation of medications altogether.
  - Lowering the dose of prednisone and increasing it when symptoms come back, trying to find the minimal effective dose. Unfortunately, frequently, when relapse occurs, the dose of prednisone will have to be increased to the highest level again and then be tapered. A small increment does not usually induce remission.
- Some patients disappear for some time before they appear again with a relapse. Recurrence may not happen immediately after the medications are discontinued, which reinforces that notion that the discontinuation of the medications is not the cause.
- Some patients do not inform their physicians that they have changed the dosage on their own, and they pretend that they do not know why the symptoms came back.
- Compliance is usually improved after one or two relapses, which make the patient more serious about taking the medications.
- Poor treatment compliance is more common in MG than in chronic diseases that do not usually respond completely to treatment, such as CIDP. The residual symptoms act as a reminder that treatment must continue.
- The need for frequent PRN courses of steroids usually leads to severe chronic side effects compared to an initially high dose followed by tapering to a low maintenance dose.
- It is possible that a PRN use of steroids makes the disease less responsive to high dose steroids when needed for exacerbations.
- Confidence of patients in their physicians may improve compliance.

REFERENCE

Dunand MB, et al. Unsatisfactory outcomes in myasthenia gravis: influence by care providers. *J Neurol.* 2010 Mar;257(3):338–343.

CASE 7.12B: THE PATIENT IN CASE 7.12A AFTER TREATMENT

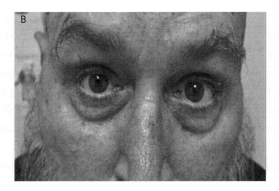

VIDEO 7.12B

The symptoms were reversed after 2 months of steroids therapy.

The next step in management is to:

1. Start azathioprine
2. Taper prednisone
3. Start mycophenolate
4. Discuss thymectomy
5. Discontinue pyridostigmine

DIAGNOSIS

- EMG was done in the hospital and revealed denervation of the tongue and upper extremities muscles and thoracic paraspinal muscles.
- AChR antibody titer is about 90% specific for MG. False positive mild elevation is reported in patients with
  - Thymoma without MG
  - Family history of MG
  - Exposure to snake toxin
  - ALS
- The patient in this case met the diagnostic criteria of ALS and the course of the disease was as expected for ALS. The presence of AChR antibodies did not change the prognosis.
- These antibodies suggest neuromuscular junction involvement in ALS. Decremental response occurs in 15% of ALS patients due to dysfunction of presynaptic calcium channels.
- Although antibody titer is usually below 0.5, titer as high as 50 nmol/L nm are reported in ALS.

REFERENCES

Okuyama Y, Mizuno T, Inoue H, Kimoto K. Amyotrophic lateral sclerosis with anti-acetylcholine receptor antibody. *Intern Med*. 1997 Apr;36(4):312–315.

Mittag T, et al. False positive immunoassay for acetylcholine receptor antibody in ALS. *NEJM*. 1980;302:868.

CHAPTER 8

DYSPHONIA

CASE 8.1: FLUCTUATING NASAL SPEECH

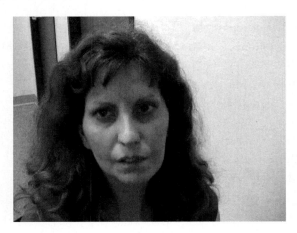

VIDEO 8.1

A 24-year-old woman presented with a 9-month history of gradually increasing and fluctuating nasal speech and regurgitation of water through her nose. Her soft palate was restricted and tongue and facial muscles were weak. Repetitive nerve stimulation (RNS) test, Tensilon test, AChR antibody titer, and computed tomography (CT) scan of the chest were non-contributory.

The most specific and appropriate next test is:

1. MuSK antibody titer
2. Single fiber electromyogram (EMG)
3. Repeat CT chest
4. Repeat RNS test
5. None of the above

DIAGNOSIS

- MuSK antibody test was positive.
- This form of autoimmune MG accounts for 40%–70% of AChR-Ab negative MG (AChR-Ab MG).
- Rarely both AChR-Ab MG and MuSK-MG coexist.
- MuSK enhances aggregation of ACh in the microtubules.
- Mostly present at age 30–50.
- 80% of patients are females.
- Onset is usually subacute.
- Dysarthria and dysphonia are universal.
- Dropped head syndrome due to weak neck extensors is common.
- Atrophy of pharyngeal muscles and tongue is common in chronic cases leading to diagnostic confusion with amyotrophic lateral sclerosis (ALS). Even tongue fasciculations were reported.
- Respiratory failure is common and myasthenic crisis is more frequent than AChR Ab MG.
- It rarely starts with extraocular muscles weakness.
- Positive RNS and thymic hyperplasia are uncommon.
- Positive Tensilon test is less likely than AChR Ab MG.
- Unlike AChR Ab MG, severity of MuSK Ab MG correlates with MuSK-Ab titer.
- Thymectomy may not be effective and is not routinely indicated.
- It is less responsive to pyridostigmine, steroids, and intravenous immunoglobulin (IVIG) and is more responsive to plasmapheresis and rituximab.
- In our experience, rituximab may induce long-term remission in refractory cases.

CASE 8.2: FAMILIAL HOARSENESS AND FOOT DROP

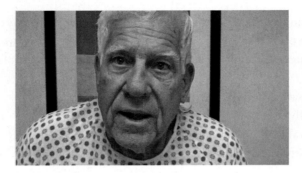

VIDEO 8.2

A 78-year-old man presented with a 7-year history of slowly progressive hoarseness and pain-less bilateral foot drop. He had mild proximal leg weakness. There was no dysphagia or ptosis. Creatine kinase (CK) level was 400 U/L and EMG showed 30% short duration units in the proximal and distal leg muscles. A twin brother developed similar signs. Muscle biopsy revealed nonspecific myopathic features with several red-rimmed vacuoles.

The most likely diagnosis is:

1. Oculopharyngeal muscular dystrophy
2. Myotilinopathy
3. Dysferlinopathy
4. Calpainopathy
5. Cavuolinopathy

DIAGNOSIS

- LGMD 1A is an autosomal dominant limb girdle muscular dystrophy caused by mutation of myotilin on chromosome 5.
- Myotilin is a sarcolemma protein that is important for the integrity of the cell membrane function.
- 50% of cases have no family history.
- Onset is usually at age 40–70 years.
- Weakness, myalgia, and hoarseness are common.
- Wrist flexion weakness and ankle extensor weakness occur with disease progression.
- Dropped head syndrome occurs in some patients, as does facial weakness.
- Dysarthria, dysphonia, and nasal speech occur in 30% of cases.
- Cardiomyopathy occurs in 50% of cases.
- Progression is slow.
- Creatine kinase (CK) is commonly two times higher than normal.
- EMG usually shows irritative myopathy.
- Muscle biopsy usually shows rimmed and autophagic vacuoles.
- Distal weakness with dysphonia is also seen in Charcot-Marie-Tooth disease types 2C, 2K, and 4A. EMG/NCS is usually enough to sort out the neuropathic from myopathic syndromes.
- Muscle biopsy is indicated for the diagnosis. If myotilin histoimmunochemistry is normal, one will have to look for a similar disorder called distal myopathy with vocal cord and pharyngeal weakness (MPD2).
  - MPD2 is an autosomal dominant disease that is reported in North America and Bulgaria and is caused by mutation of a nuclear gene called Martin 3 (MATR 3) on chromosome 5q31.2.
  - Average age of onset is 46 years, and weakness starts in the distal anterior leg muscle (foot drop) and sometimes spreads to the arms.
  - Voice is affected in 65% of cases and usually occurs after limb weakness.
  - Dysphagia is common.
  - Serum CK: normal to 8 times normal.
  - EMG: Chronic myopathic changes.
  - Muscle pathology: nonspecific chronic myopathic changes, rare rimmed vacuoles.
  - MATR 3: variable staining of myonuclei.

CASE 8.3: CHRONIC NASAL SPEECH

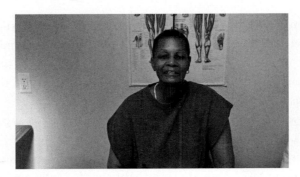

VIDEO 8.3

A 46-year-old woman presented with a 10-year history of speech and swallowing difficulty. Her neck extensors were 4/5 and extraocular movements were full. There was a mild tongue weakness. There was no ptosis. Symptoms consistently became worse in the evenings and when she was tired. There were times when her symptoms became very mild. AChR antibody titer was negative. EMG revealed no proximal myopathic abnormalities. RNS test and CT chest were normal. Brian MRI was normal. She did not respond to pyridostigmine.

The most reasonable next step is to test for:

1. MuSK antibody associated MG
2. Diphtheria
3. Kennedy disease
4. Hypoglossal palsy
5. Brainstem glioma

DIAGNOSIS

- MuSK MG is more common in females and mostly affects the pharyngeal muscles.
- It can go undetected for years due to negative AChR antibodies and the lack of ocular symptoms.
- Atrophy of pharyngeal muscles and even tongue fasciculations are reported, leading to misdiagnosis as ALS.
- Response to pyridostigmine, prednisone, and thymectomy is not as good as in AChR Ab associated MG.
- Plasmaphoresis and rituximab are reported to be effective when other measures fail.
- Rare cases of ocular MG are reported in association with MuSK antibodies.
- Double positive serology is also reported.

CASE 8.4: VOCAL CORD PARALYSIS AND DISTAL WEAKNESS

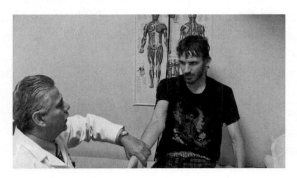

VIDEO 8.4

A 31-year-old man presented with hands and feet numbness since he was 8 years old. Gradually he developed ataxia, and distal arm and leg weakness and loss of reflexes. He also developed hoarseness. Cerebrospinal fluid (CSF) protein was 50 mg/dl with normal cells. NCS revealed the following: peroneal and tibial motor conduction velocities of 34–35m/sec and compound muscle action potential (CMAP) amplitudes of 1 mv with distal motor latencies of 8–9 msec and prolonged F responses. Sural responses were absent and he had bilateral focal ulnar slowing at the elbows. EMG was normal. Ear, nose, and throat (ENT) evaluation revealed vocal cord paralysis. He was treated with intravenous immunoglobulin (IVIG) for 8 months with no improvement. His mother had similar symptoms. He had high feet arches. Testing for CMT type 1A was negative.

These association is typically seen in:

1. Chronic inflammatory demyelinating polyneuropathy (CIDP)
2. Charcot-Marie-Tooth (CMT) 2D
3. CMT 4B
4. CMT 4A
5. CMT 4E

DIAGNOSIS

- Combination of vocal cord paralysis and distal weakness is seen in LGMD 1A (myotilin-opathy) and in CMT 2C, 2K and 4A.
- CMT 2C: autosomal dominant axonal neuropathy due to mutation of TRPV4 gene on chromosome 12.
- CMT2K is due to GDAP1 protein mutation on Chromosome 8 q21.11 and has several phenotypes.
  - ◆ Axonal, recessive
  - ◆ Axonal, dominant
  - ◆ Recessive, intermediate A (CMT RIA)
    - ▪ It presents in early childhood with gait imbalance and causes distal sensory loss and proximal and distal weakness. Nerve conduction study (NCS) shows mixed demyelinating and axonal features. Nerve pathology shows mixed axonal and demyelinating features.
- CMT 4A: GDAP1 mutation, same gene as CMT 2K
  - ◆ Usually starts before 2 years of age
  - ◆ Progressive, distal weakness, vocal cord paralysis, and absent reflexes
  - ◆ Motor conduction slowing and low CMAP amplitudes
  - ◆ Pathology is mostly demyelinating
- Ganglioside-induced differentiation-associated protein 1 is a protein that in humans is encoded by the *GDAP1* gene.
  - ◆ This gene encodes a member of the ganglioside-induced differentiation-associated protein family, which may play a role in a signal transduction pathway during neuronal development. Mutations in this gene have been associated with various forms of Charcot-Marie-Tooth disease.

CHAPTER 9

DYSPNEA

CASE 9.1: BREATHING DIFFICULTY AND INVOLUNTARY MOVEMENT

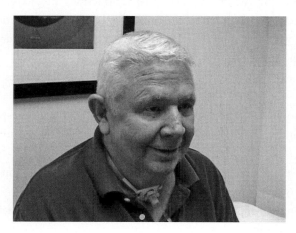

VIDEO 9.1

A 67-year-old man presented with a 10-year history of breathing difficulty. This disorder may be associated with:

1. Blepharospasm
2. Dysphagia
3. Airway obstruction
4. Spasmodic dysphonia
5. All of the above

DIAGNOSIS

- The examination showed involuntary facial contractions, blepharospasm, and bursts of breathing difficulty that seemed to be caused by laryngeal contractions. These findings are consistent with oromandibular dystonia. Other features include dysphagia, airway obstruction, and spasmodic dysphonia.
- Patients with dystonia may be referred to neuromuscular clinics due to respiratory problems.
- Movement disorders may be associated with different patterns of respiratory disorders.
  - Upper respiratory tract obstruction and/or diaphragmatic dysfunction are the main ones.
- Spasmodic dysphonia may also cause upper airway obstruction. Sometimes the respiratory difficulty is severe enough to mandate a tracheostomy.
- The most common symptoms are stridor, gasping, dyspnea, and interrupted speech and paradoxical breathing.
- In this patient with craniocervical dystonia, the involuntary contraction of the posterior pharyngeal muscles and upper respiratory airways was associated with a paradoxical contraction of the vocalis muscles, mostly during inspiration, and the vocal cord adduction caused gasping.
- Desynchronized contraction of the diaphragm, chest, and upper respiratory airway muscles leads to dyspnea.

REFERENCE

Mehanna R, Jankovic J. Respiratory problems in neurologic movement disorders. *Parkinsonism Related Disorders*. 2010;16:628–638.

CASE 9.2: RESPIRATORY FAILURE AND POSITIVE FSDH DELETION

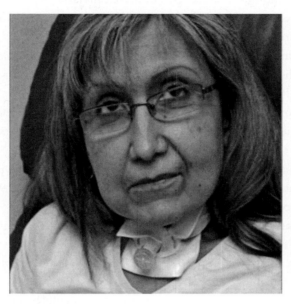

VIDEO 9.2

A 56-year-old woman presented with recurrent prolonged respiratory failure after viral upper respiratory tract infection at least once a year. Creatine kinase (CK) level was 420 U/L. Electromyogram (EMG) repeatedly showed myopathic units with fibrillations in the proximal arm and leg muscles and paraspinal muscles. Nerve conduction study (NCS) was normal. Arterial blood gase (ABG) analysis revealed hypercapnia and pulmonary function test (PFT) showed a restrictive pattern. Muscle biopsy showed only type II fiber atrophy and diaphragmatic biopsy showed mild inflammation. She responded partially and temporarily to oral steroids and intravenous immunoglobulin (IVIG). There was no facial weakness or scapular winging but mild pectoralis atrophy. Dry spot for acid alpha glucosidase (GGA) revealed normal activity. Facioscapulohumeral muscular dystrophy (FSHD) mutation analysis was positive for D4Z4 allel contraction.

The positive FSHD mutation in this case:

1. Is 100% specific
2. Should be confirmed by looking for a distal permissive gene
3. Is consistent with the typical clinical picture of FSHD
4. Should be confirmed by mutation analysis on muscle tissue

DIAGNOSIS

- FSHD is one of the most common genetic muscle diseases.
- Facial weakness, scapular winging, asymmetrical foot drop, and proximal weakness are common features.
- Respiratory compromise occurs very late in the course and usually after the extremities weakness has become severe. Otherwise, respiratory compromise is so rare that its presence should call for reconsideration of the diagnosis.
- Genetic diagnosis of FSHD is based on identification of partial deletion of a large repetitive DNA element known as D4Z4 and is present in the subtelomeric region of chromosome 4q.
  - Each D4Z4 repeat is 3.3 Kb in size, and normal individuals typically have 10–100 D4Z4 repeats on each copy of chromosome 4q. In greater than 95% of patients with FSHD, one copy of the 4q will have only 1–9 repeats.
  - Deletion of an integral number of D4Z4 repeats is necessary but not sufficient to cause FSHD.
  - Contraction must occur on the A variant (4qA) (Figure 9.2.1) in order for the D4Z4 mutation to be pathogenic.
- In atypical cases of FSHD, a positive deletion of D4Z4 should be supplemented by testing for the A variant.
- In this case, myopathies with respiratory failure as a common feature should be considered in the differential diagnosis such as:
  1. Adult onset nemaline myopathy
  2. Myofibrillar myopathies
  3. Acid maltase deficiency
  4. Calpainopathy
  5. Amyloid myopathy
  6. Inflammatory myopathies

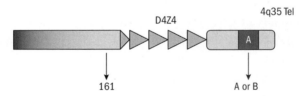

FIGURE 9.2.1 (A) variant (distal permissive gene) is essential for the diagnosis of FSHD. *Courtesy of Rabi Tawil, MD.*

CASE 9.3: PERSISTENT RESPIRATORY FAILURE AFTER A CAR ACCIDENT

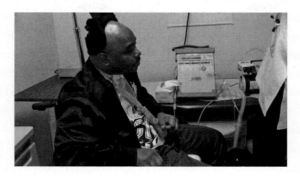

VIDEO 9.3

A 50-year-old man developed breathing difficulty after a car accident, which progressed to respiratory failure that required a tracheostomy. While in a long-term facility, his creatine kinase (CK) was found to be around 1900 U/L repeatedly. His examination revealed mild proximal weakness. EMG showed proximal myopathic units with spontaneous paraspinal discharges. Muscle biopsy showed normal glycogen contents. Muscle and blood tissue acid alpha glucosidase (GAA) activity was low. GAA sequence analysis confirmed mutation of GAA gene. He improved slightly with GAA infusions.

The following are typical for this case except:

1. Predominant respiratory involvement
2. Irritative myopathy
3. Positive response to GAA
4. Low GAA activity in blood and muscle
5. Normal glycogen content in the muscle

DIAGNOSIS

- Among the myopathies that affect respiratory muscles early and out of proportion to the extremities and bulbar muscles, acid maltase deficiency is the most important.
- 30% of cases present with respiratory failure that is usually triggered by infection.
- Headache, sleepiness, orthopnea, and dyspnea are common presenting features.
- All patients develop respiratory failure during evolution of the disease.
- The enzyme is a lysosomal housekeeper that is widely distributed in the tissue.
- In adult form, the enzyme activity is hugely reduced in muscle and white cells.
- Severity of disease correlates with enzyme activity.
- Autosomal recessive, 17q23. Incidence: 2:100,000.
- Age: 10–60 years with history of muscle cramps, fatigue, mild muscle weakness for years.
- Expiration is more affected than inspiration, leading to weak cough and atelectasis.
- Weakness is more proximal than distal. Scapular winging may lead to confusion with FSHD.
- Cardiomyopathy is common.
- EMG: irritative myopathy and paraspinal myotonic discharges.
- CK can be normal in adults.
- Muscle biopsy: glycogen in cytoplasm and lysosomal vacuoles (positive acid phosphatase).
- Less glycogen deposition is seen in adults than in infantile and juvenile forms, and atypically, cases of no glycogen accumulation may still show abnormal GAA activity.
- If clinically and electromyographically suspected, a dry blood spot is recommended.
- Intravenous recombinant alpha glucosidase is shown to improve strength, especially in young population.
- Debrancher enzyme deficiency should be considered if GAA activity is normal. It can cause similar clinical and EMG pictures.

CASE 9.4: DYSPNEA AND SCAPULAR WINGING

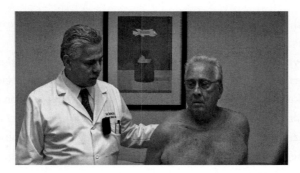

VIDEO 9.4

A 65-year-old man presented with acute right arm pain and dyspnea. Cervical magnetic resonance imaging (MRI) and brachial plexus MRI were normal. EMG showed denervation of the right rhomboid and diaphragm.

The most likely diagnosis is:

1. Parsonage turner syndrome
2. C3-C5 radiculopathy
3. Mononeuritis multiplex
4. Scapuloperoneal neuropathy
5. HNPP

DIAGNOSIS

- The acute and painful onset and the involvement of the dorsal scapular, axillary, and phrenic nerves suggest neuralgic amyotrophy.
- Neuralgic amyotrophy is a rare autoimmune inflammation of the brachial plexus.
- Sudden and severe burning pain in the shoulder and periscapular region for few days, followed by weakness and atrophy of certain arm muscles, depending on the affected nerves.
- A similar syndrome affaecting the lumbar plexus is reported. Thrity percent of cases are bilateral. A hereditary variant called hereditary neuralgic amyotrophy exists.
- Before weakness becomes obvious, the condition may be misdiagnosed as a shoulder arthritis, or herpes zoster.
- After weakness appears, other diagnoses are considered, such as cervical HNP, tumor of the spinal cord or brachial plexus, and thoracic outlet syndrome.
- Axillary, suprascapular, long thoracic, and musculocutaneous nerves are most commonly affected. Radial, anterior interosseus, median, ulnar, and phrenic nerves are next in frequency.
- Steroids provide no benefit but may reduce pain and enhance tolerance to physical therapy.
- Pain management and rehabilitation are the mainstay of treatment. Most patients recover within 2 years with minimal residual deficit.

CHAPTER 10

WEAKNESS OF THE NECK MUSCLES

CASE 10.1: INABILITY TO HOLD HEAD UP

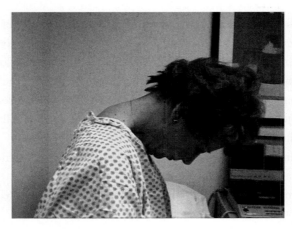

VIDEO 10.1

A 59-year-old woman presented with pain and fatigability of neck extension evolved over 3 months. She soon developed slurring of speech and choking, especially in the evenings. Her examination showed weakness of the neck extensors and tongue atrophy with hyperreflexia.

Dropped head syndrome is a recognized manifestation of all the following except:

1. MuSK myasthenia gravis (MG)
2. Amyotrophic lateral sclerosis (ALS)
3. Facioscapulohumeral muscular dystrophy (FSHD)
4. Polymyositis
5. Myotonia congenita

DIAGNOSIS

- The ability to hold the head up is made possible by at least 5 pairs of neck extensor muscles. It is a function that is taken for granted until it becomes defective.
- An average human head weighs 9 pounds. Animals have more developed neck extensors.
- Weakness of the neck extensors initially leads to inability to lift the head off the pillow; therefore the patient has to turn to the side before sitting up. With progression, it becomes hard to hold the head up for a long time, and then the head drops all the time so that the patient has to hold his chin up with hands to be able to see.
- Excessive strain on the neck extensors leads to posterior cervical pain, which is a common early manifestation.
- The affected muscles appear atrophic, edematous, and are replaced by fat, as demonstrated by cervical magnetic resonance imaging (MRI).
- Common causes of dropped head syndrome:
  1. ALS: weakness of the neck extensors is usually accompanied by bulbar dysfunction (dysphagia, dysarthria, dyspnea) and features of upper motor neuron (UMN) and lower motor neuron (LMN) lesions are seen. It is progressive, and diagnosis is hardly difficult. Mild creatine kinase (CK) elevation may deceivingly sway the diagnosis toward a myopathic process, but widespread denervation is usually evident by electromyogram (EMG).
  2. Myasthenia gravis (MG): usually fatigable diplopia and ptosis are present. In MuSK MG, dysphagia, fluctuating dysarthria, and tongue weakness and atrophy may lead to diagnostic confusion with ALS, which also shows decremental response in about 30% of times. Even tongue fasciculations are reported in cases with MuSK MG. It is strongly recommended that MuSK antibodies are tested in patients with dropped head syndrome.
  3. Inflammatory myopathies
  4. Metabolic myopathies such as acid maltase deficiency
  5. Adult onset nemaline myopathy with monoclonal gammopathy
  6. FSHD
  7. Dystrophic myopathies like dysferlinopathy
  8. Chronic inflammatory demyelinating polyneuropathy (CIDP)
- After extensive evaluation, at least 25% of neck extensor weakness remains idiopathic (isolated neck extensors myopathy; INEM).
- There are reports of response of INEM to immunomodulation. Some cases may represent restricted seronegative myasthenia, while others may represent restricted muscular dystrophy or axial myopathy (Muppidi S, et al., 2010).
- The finding of spontaneous activity in the cervical paraspinal muscles should not be over-interpreted. These changes can be secondary to the head drop and not primary.

REFERENCE

Muppidi S, et al. Isolated neck extensor myopathy: is it responsive to immunotherapy? *J Clin Neuromuscl Dis.* 2010 Sep;12(1):26–29.

CASE 10.2: SPOTTING MONEY IN THE POST OFFICE

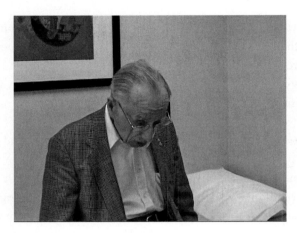

VIDEO 10.2

A 75-year-old man developed difficulty holding his head up that had been noticed a year earlier. There was no pain, diplopia, or ptosis. He had mild weakness of the hip flexors and fatigable weakness of the neck extensors. He told a story about a friend who spotted a lot of money since she developed a similar syndrome. Repetitive left spinal accessory nerve stimulation revealed a 15% decremental response of the left trapezius.

The most specific test for a treatable cause of dropped head syndrome is:

1. Muscle biopsy
2. FSHD mutation analysis
3. AChR antibodies
4. Repetitive nerve stimulation (RNS)
5. Striational antibodies

DIAGNOSIS

- This gentleman was joking about a friend who spotted money many times in the post office during the Christmas season due to the fact that she had to look down all the time as she had a dropped head.
- Investigations on this patient revealed a very high AChR antibody titer. He responded well to prednisone.

The following investigations are appropriate in patients with dropped head syndrome:

1. Creatine kinase (CK) activity: marked elevation would suggest a myopathic process while mild elevation would be consistent with a neurogenic etiology.
2. Immunofixation protein electrophoresis (IFPE): monoclonal gammopathy would suggest an adult onset nemaline myopathy. However, monoclonal gammopathy can be normal in the elderly.
3. EMG to look for widespread denervation, which would suggest motor neuron disease, and to look for signs of irritative myopathy.
4. MRI of the cervical and thoracic paraspinal muscles to look for edematous and fatty changes.
5. Muscle biopsy: in the absence of peripheral muscles weakness and with normal CK and EMG, the utility of a muscle biopsy is questionable. Biopsy of paraspinal muscles has its limitations; in addition, these muscles are not standardized and their normal histology is not well characterized.
6. In the absence of neuromuscular etiology, a referral to a movement disorder clinic would be appropriate to rule out other causes such as Parkinson disease, anterocollis, and multisystem atrophy.

CASE 10.3: BENT NECK

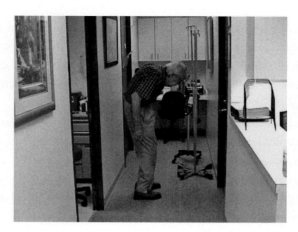

VIDEO 10.3

A 76-year-old man developed gait instability and abnormal head posture gradually over 10 years. He had no diplopia, dysphagia, or leg weakness. When he lay flat, his spine was fully extended. MG serology was negative. EMG revealed restricted thoracic and cervical spontaneous discharges (fibrillations and positive sharp waves).

The most likely diagnosis is:

1. Camptocormia
2. Myasthenia gravis (MG)
3. Amyotrophic lateral sclerosis (ALS)
4. Spine disorder
5. Parkinson disease (PD)

DIAGNOSIS

- Camptocormia is derived from Greek *kamptos* (bend) and *kormos* (trunk). It refers to abnormal posture dure to hyperflexion of the thoraco-lumbar spines, which is relieved in the recumbent position, thus differing from those caused by spinal deformities. Early in the course, it becomes progressively difficult to maintain erect orthostatic posture. Later, the thoracolumbar flexion becomes fixed during walking.

- For decades, camptocormia was considered to be psychogenic because it was assumed by soldiers who could not cope with the stress of the World War I and II; it may have been triggered by stooped posture while walking in the trenches.

- More recent studies revealed many causes for camptocormia:
  - Movement disorders such as PD and dystonia. This patient had a normal arm swing and facial expression.
  - Neuromuscular disorders: discussed in case 10.2; mostly include ALS, MG, and dystrophic, and inflammatory myopathies
  - Spinal deformities
  - Psychogenic disorders

- Those associated with PD may respond to botulinum toxin injection to the abdominal and neck muscles.

- Fatty infiltration of the paraspinal muscles would support a myopathic etiology.

- EMG is usually helpful to differentiate between a central and peripheral etiology. However, paraspinal fibrillations and positive sharp waves can be secondary to abnormal posture and if restricted do not have to imply a primary myopathic process.

- Like the case with INEM, many cases of camptocormia remain idiopathic. *Idiopathic thoracic extensor myopathy* (ITEM) is a term coined by Richard Barohn, MD, who speculated that ITEM is a senile degenerative process of the thoracic paraspinal muscles. No treatment is available.

REFERENCE

Shinjo SK, et al. Camptocormia: a rare axial myopathy disease. *Clinics*. 2008 June;63(3):416–417.

CASE 10.4: PROGRESSIVE HEAD DROP

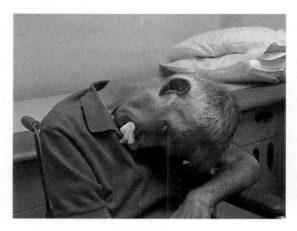

VIDEO 10.4

A 65-year-old man presented with progressive weakness of the neck extensors, dysarthria, dysphagia, and hypersialosis, developed over a year. He was hyperreflexic and his tongue showed atrophy and fasciculations. He expired 3 months after this video.

The most likely cause of dropped head syndrome in this case is:

1. Spinal muscular atrophy
2. Primary lateral sclerosis
3. Amyotrophic lateral sclerosis (ALS)
4. Myasthenia gravis (MG)
5. Parkinson disease (PD)

DIAGNOSIS

- In less than 2% of ALS patients, weakness of the neck extensors is an early and the presenting feature of ALS.
- It is attributed to preferential degeneration of the motor neurons controlling the paraspinal muscles.
- These patients usually develop bulbar dysfunction early, and they may have a worse prognosis.
- The diagnosis of ALS is hardly a problem in these patients who usually have clear upper and lower motor neuron signs at the time of presentation.
- Dropped head causes social embarrassment and increased morbidity and it interferes with cough, clearing of secretions, and eating.
- Hard cervical collar may help, but temporarily, and most patients find it inconvenient.
- An old method using a back stick, an abdominal belt, and a forehead band is employed by some patients.
- As the disease progresses, the dropped head, along with the wasting and weakness of the extremities muscles, renders the patient totally invalid.
- This patient continued to fight despite the terminal nature of his illness. He died from chest infection.
- Providing terminal care to ALS patients is a challenge to the patients and their heathcare providers and it lacks universally acceptable guidelines.

REFERENCE

Gourie-Devi M, Nalini A, Sandhya S. Early or late appearance of "dropped head syndrome" in amyotrophic lateral sclerosis. *J Neurol Neurosurg Psychiatry*. 2003;74:683–686. doi:10.1136/jnnp.74.5.683.

CASE 10.5A, B: DROPPED HEAD
AND CHEWING DIFFICULTY

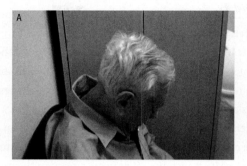

VIDEO 10.5A

An 83-year-old man developed the shown clinical picture over a month.

The most likely cause of this dropped head syndrome is:

1. Amyotrophic lateral sclerosis (ALS)
2. Myasthenia gravis (MG)
3. Lambert-Eaton syndrome
4. Polymyositis
5. Guillain-Barré syndrome

DIAGNOSIS

- Weak neck extensor muscles can be the initial manifestation of MG, but usually it develops with other ocular and bulbar symptoms such as diplopia, ptosis, dysarthria, dysphagia, dyspnea, and fatigability of the chewing muscles.
- It is imperative to test fatigability of neck extensors in all myasthenics, even if they do not complain of weakness of these muscles. Increased fatigability of the neck extensors and triceps muscle is often used to differentiate MG from myopathies where weakness usually affects neck flexors and deltoid.
- One has to be careful when performing repetitive neck flexion/extension testing in the elderly with severe cervical spondylosis and patients with a history of neck trauma.
- Dropped head due to MG is usually not as pronounced in the mornings.
- MuSK antibodies associated MG may present with dropped head as the main feature.
- The lack of ocular involvement and the atrophy of the tongue and pharynx may lead to diagnostic confusion with ALS.
- Dysarthria is not a differentiating feature as it occurs in both.
- Measurement of MuSK Ab is important in all cases of dropped head syndrome.
- A therapeutic steroid trial may be warranted in uncertain cases.
- Weakness and fatigability of neck extensors usually start improving within 3 weeks of initiation of steroids.
- Dropped head due to MG usually responds well to treatment of MG. This patient was placed on plasmapheresis and oral prednisone and his symptoms resolved within 2 months (Video 10.5B).

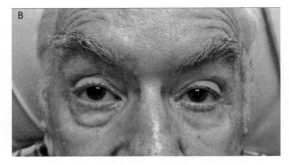

VIDEO 10.5B

CASE 10.6: NO MORE THAN DROPPED HEAD

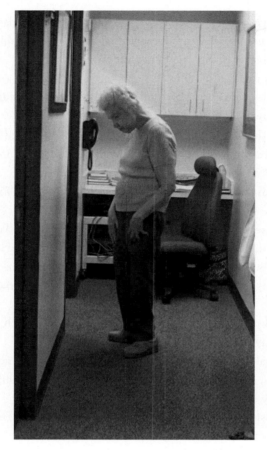

VIDEO 10.6

A 79-year-old woman presented with a 12-month history of neck discomfort and an abnormal stance. She had no proximal extremity weakness, dysphagia, dysarthria, diplopia, or ptosis. CK level was normal. AChR antibody test was negative. EMG of the extremities revealed no myopathic units. EMG of cervical and thoracic paraspinal muscles showed fibs and positive sharp waves. Repetitive nerve stimulation test was normal. MRI of the cervical and thoracic spines revealed atrophy and fatty replacement of the paraspinal muscles.

This is most likely a case of:

1. Isolated neck extensor myopathy (INEM)
2. Myasthenia gravis (MG)
3. Polymyositis
4. Amyotrophic lateral sclerosis (ALS)
5. Camptocormia

DIAGNOSIS

- Dropped head syndrome can be caused by many neuromuscular disorders and sometimes it is the presenting feature of these disorders, which could be myopathic, myasthenic, neuropathic, and motor neuronopathic.
- Sometimes weakness continues to be restricted to the cervical and sometimes thoracic paraspinal muscles, and evaluation fails to reveal a cause. This entity is called isolated neck extensors myopathy (INEM).
- It usually affects the elderly population and presents with dropped head and kyphosis due to weakness and atrophy of the thoracic paraspinal muscles. Gait abnormality to adjust for the axial weakness is common.
- Posture is normal during supine position, unlike patients with fixed contracture of the spines.
- Some of these cases are familial, while others are due to restricted muscular dystrophy or myopathy (axial myopathy).
- CK level is usually normal and EMG may show myopathic units in the paraspinal muscles with spontaneous activity. Paraspinal muscle biopsy usually shows nonspecific myopathic findings.
- These EMG and pathologic findings should be interpreted with caution since most of these changes may be secondary to the altered head position.
- Rarely, paraspinal muscle biopsy shows specific findings like nemaline rods or many ragged red fibers, suggesting adult onset nemaline myopathy and mitochondrial disorders, respectively.
- Immunosuppression (e.g., steroids with or without azathioprine) is shown to be effective in some of these cases and is worth a trial.
- This case did improve with azathioprine.

REFERENCE

Muppidi S, Saperstein DS, Shaibani A, Nations SP, Vernino S, Wolfe GI. Isolated neck extensor myopathy: is it responsive to immunotherapy? *J Clin Neuromuscul Dis.* 2010 Sep;12(1):26–29.

CASE 10.7: A TWISTED NECK AFTER BIRTH

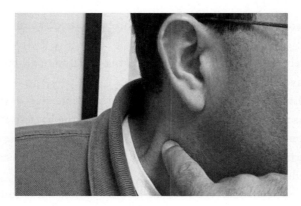

VIDEO 10.7

A 32-year-old man was born with forceps assistance and had multiple head and neck hematomas. As he grew up, he developed a head tilt to the left. Examination is shown.

This is most likely a case of head tilt as:

1. Cervical dystonia
2. Congenital torticollis
3. Axial myopathy
4. Cervical tic
5. Bad habit

DIAGNOSIS

- Abnormal head tilt can be a cause of referral to neuromuscular clinics due to suspicion of weakness.
- Weakness rarely leads to lateral tilt of the head but may lead to dropped head.
- Torticollis may be divided into:
  1. Congenital muscular torticollis, which is due to birth injury of the sternocleidomastoid (SCM) muscles resulting in fibrosis and turning of the head to the side of the weak muscles. Sometimes this leads to deformity of the face, base of the skull, and cranium. Most of the time, it resolves spontaneously in few years. Otherwise, surgical myotomy may be needed.
  2. Spasmodic torticollis: this is also called cervical dystonia. It is due to hyperactive cervical muscles. The head is turned away from the hyperactive muscle. It responds to botulinum toxin.
  3. Ocular torticollis: weakness of the extraocular muscles (EOM) leads to a corrective head tilt. Weak superior oblique leads to a head tilt away from the affected side. There is no restriction of the cervical motion otherwise.

CASE 10.8: DROPPED HEAD AND RIGIDITY

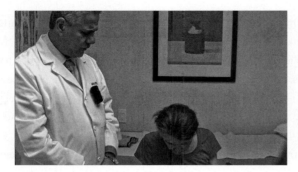

VIDEO 10.8

A 71-year-old woman presented with a 2-month history of difficulty walking and lifting her head. Her examination revealed normal neck extensors strength, cogwheeling, hypophonia, and hypomimia.

The most likely cause of dropped head in this case is:

1. Amyotrophic lateral sclerosis (ALS)
2. Parkinson disease (PD)
3. Myasthenia gravis (MG)
4. Isolated neck extensor myopathy
5. Camptocormia

DIAGNOSIS

- The most common cause of dropped head in the neuromuscular clinic is weakness of the neck extensors due to neuromuscular disorders such as myopathies, MG, and ALS.
- Some patients who are referred to the neuromuscular clinic do not have weakness of the neck extensors, and the cause of the drop is dystonia of the neck flexors and abdominal muscles.
- Dropped head syndrome is common in multisystem atrophy and rare in Parkinson disease.
- Although it is mostly a chronic condition, acute deterioration has been reported.
- Response to anti-parkinsonian medications is not consistent. Botulinum toxin is reported to be effective if injected to the neck flexors and abdominal muscles.

REFERENCE

Kashihara K, et al. Dropped head in Parkinson disease. *Mov Disord.* 2006 Aug;21(8):1213–1216.

CASE 10.9: DROPPED HEAD

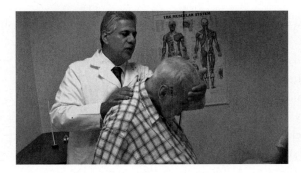

VIDEO 10.9

A 69-year-old man presented with a 6-month history of posterior neck pain during walking. He then could not hold his head up and had mild left ptosis and horizontal diplopia that resolved when he closed one eye.

Examination is shown.

The most specific and appropriate diagnostic test in this case is:

1. RNS
2. AChR antibody titer
3. EMG
4. Muscle biopsy
5. MRI of the cervical spines

DIAGNOSIS

- Dropped head syndrome is due to weakness of neck extensors or dystonia of the neck flexors.
- Examination demonstrated weakness of the neck extensors.
- The most common neuromuscula causes are:
  - ◆ Amyotrophic lateral sclerosis
  - ◆ Myopathies
  - ◆ Isolated neck extensor myopathy
  - ◆ MG: this is suggested by diplopia and ptosis
- The most specific test is AChR antibody titer.
- Prognosis of MG is good, and most patients regain full strength within 3 months of treatment.

CHAPTER 11

SCAPULAR WINGING

CASE 11.1: SCAPULAR WINGING AND LOBULATED FIBERS

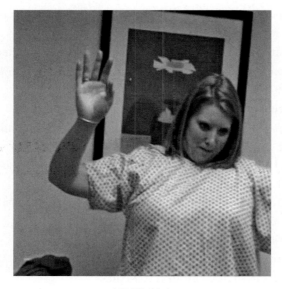

VIDEO 11.1

A 30-year-old woman presented with a slowly progressive arm weakness that started 7 years earlier. In addition to what is shown, she had mild facial weakness. There was no family history of muscle disease. Creatine kinase (CK) level was 350 U/L, electromyogram (EMG) revealed 30% short duration polyphasic units in the periscapular muscles. Muscle biopsy is shown in Figure 11.1.1.

Facioscapulohumeral muscular dystrophy (FSHD) mutation analysis was negative.

Scapular winging in this case is most likely due to:

1. Limb girdle muscular dystrophy (LGMD) 2A (calpainopathy)
2. LGMD 2B (dysferlinopathy)
3. FSHD type 2
4. Scapuloperoneal syndrome
5. Polymyositis

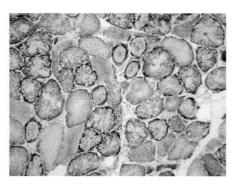

FIGURE 11.1.1 NADH-TR reaction, 100x.

DIAGNOSIS

- Muscle biopsy revealed active myopathy with many lobulated fibers.
- Calpain-3 is a mostly calcium-dependent and muscle-specific enzyme that is important for cytoskeletal modeling. Its exact function is not clear.
- More than 60 pathogenic mutations of calpain-3 have been identified.
- It is the most common LGMD and affects children and adults (25% of dystrophies with normal dystrophin and sarcoglycans).
- The clinical picture may mimic FSHD due to scapular winging.
- It usually affects hamstrings and thighs adductors early. MRI confirmation of preferential involvement of these muscles is diagnostically helpful.
- Periscapular and humeral muscles are usually affected a few years after onset.
- Distal and facial muscles are usually spared, unlike FSHD.
- Early elbow and calf contractures may lead to misdiagnosis of EDMD.
- 50% of patients are nonambulatory by age 20.
- No cardiac, intellectual, or respiratory involvement is expected.
- Longevity is normal.
- 6% of patients have asymptomatic hyperCKemia.
- CK is normal or up to 20x normal. EMG: myopathy with no muscle membrane irritability. Muscle biopsy: nonspecific myopathic features. Lobulated fibers are common, though nonspecific.
- Decreased enzyme activity in the muscle tissue is seen in 80% of cases (western blot confirmation is necessary).
- Genetic confirmation is necessary because secondary calpain deficiency can be seen in dysferlinopathy and titinopathy.

REFERENCE

Figarella-Branger D, et al. Myopathy with lobulated muscle fibers: evidence for heterogeneous etiology and clinical presentation. *Neuromuscul Disord*. 2002 Jan;12(1):4–12.

CASE 11.2: SCAPULAR WINGING AFTER CERVICAL LYMPH NODE BIOPSY

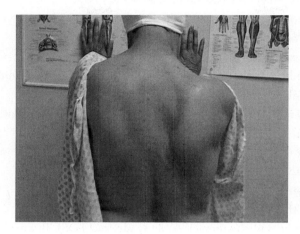

VIDEO 11.2

A 37-year-old woman who had a cervical lymph node biopsy 3 months earlier presented with pain and stiffness of the right upper back muscles that did not respond to gabapentin. She developed tingling of the right little fingers a couple of weeks earlier. A chiropractic manipulation gave her a temporary relief. Examination is shown.

EMG is expected to show denervation of:

1. Rhomboid
2. Trapezius
3. Serratus anterior
4. Levator scapulae
5. Supraspinatus

Tingling of the right little finger that developed later was most likely:

1. Not related to the scapular winging
2. Due to a related thoracic outlet syndrome
3. Due to a related focal ulnar neuropathy at the elbow
4. Due to an incidental C8 radiculopathy
5. Was associated with reduced ulnar compound muscle action potential (CMAP) amplitude

DIAGNOSIS

- The trapezius stabilizes the base of the scapula.
- It originates from the spinous processes of the cervical and thoracic vertebrae and inserts into the spine of the scapula.
- The spinal accessory nerve (SAN) branches from the 3rd and 4th cervical roots.
- Surgical procedures in the posterior triangle of the neck can cause injury to the SAN due to its superficial location in that region.
- Patients rarely notice the winged scapula and they usually present with periscapular pain and stiffness.
- Scapular winging is lateral. The scapula deviates laterally, unlike the medial winging seen in long thoracic neuropathy.
- Proximal lesion leads to sternocleidomastoid weakness as well.
- Depression of the shoulder is an important diagnostic clue.
- Shoulder droop may lead to thoracic outlet syndrome (TOS). This explains why the patient later developed little finger numbness. Typically, in neurogenic TOS there is a reduction of the ipsilateral ulnar sensory nerve action potential (SNAP) and median CMAP.
- On nerve conduction studies, stimulation of the right SAN did not produce a motor response (by comparison, the amplitude of the left CMAP was 6mV).
- Needle examination showed active denervation changes in the right trapezius. Needle EMG of the right rhomboid and serratus anterior was normal.
- Surgical options include transfer of the levator scapula to the spine of the scapula, which has been reported to result in return of function and relief of pain.
- Levator scapulae is supplied by branched from the fourth and fifth cervical nerves and frequently by a branch from the dorsal scapular nerve.

REFERENCE

Bigliani LU, Compito CA, Duralde XA, Wolfe IN. Transfer of the levator scapulae, rhomboid major, and rhomboid minor for paralysis of the trapezius. *J Bone Joint Surg Am*. 1996 Oct;78(10):1534–1540.

CASE 11.3: PROGRESSIVE SCAPULAR WINGING AND SHORTNESS OF BREATH

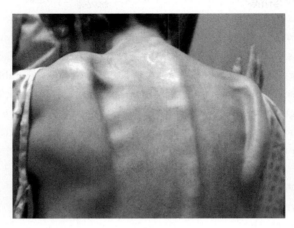

VIDEO 11.3

A 69-year-old female presented with a 6-month history of shortness of breath, weakness of the arms, and weight loss. Examination demonstrated atrophy of the periscapular muscles and winging of the scapulae, fasciculations of the arm muscles, hyperreflexia, and normal sensation. Creatine kinase (CK) level was 320 U/L. EMG showed active denervation of the proximal arm muscles and of the cervical and thoracic paraspinal muscles.

Periscapular wasting and dyspnea in this case are features of:

1. Becker muscular dystrophy (MD)
2. Motor neuron disease
3. Acid maltase deficiency
4. FSHD
5. Amyloid myopathy

DIAGNOSIS

- The scapulae play an important role in arm abduction and rotation. They are held in place by several muscles to ensure their stability during such movements.
- Scapular winging is a sign of weakness of one or more of the periscapular muscles.
- Laterally, the serratus anterior prevents the scapula from being displaced medially during arm movements. Medially, the rhomboids and trapezius muscles stabilize the scapulae.
- Lesions to these muscles or their nerve supplies may lead to scapular winging.
- Causes of winging of the scapulae:
  - Diffuse muscle disease that leads to symmetrical or asymmetrical weakness of the periscapular muscles:
    - FSHD
    - LGMD 2A
    - Emery Dreifuss muscular dystrophy
    - Desmin myopathy
    - Centronuclear myopathy
  - Diffuse denervation:
    - ALS
    - Spinal muscular atrophy (SMA), type 4
    - Scapuloperoneal syndrome
  - Focal nerve lesion:
    - Long thoracic neuropathy
    - Spinal accessory neuropathy
    - Dorsal scapular neuropathy
- While scapular winging is not usually a presenting sign in ALS, it is important to know that wasting of the periscapular muscles does occur commonly in ALS when upper limbs are involved. Scapular winging can easily be appreciated when the patient is disrobed for EMG.
- Diagnosis of ALS was suggested clinically by the presence of both upper and lower motor neuron signs. EMG findings supported the diagnosis of ALS.
- Weakness of ventilatory muscles is common in these patients. Bulbar involvement occurs soon if it is not already present by the time that periscapular wasting has occurred.
- Periscapular atrophy contributed to poor arm abduction in this case and thus compounded the patient's functional limitations.

CASE 11.4: SCAPULAR WINGING AND DEAFNESS

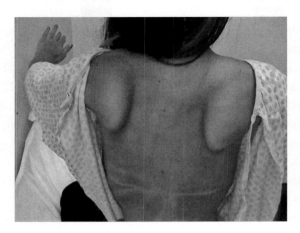

VIDEO 11.4

A 28-year-old woman presented with a 3-year history of arm weakness. She gradually developed right foot drop. Her mother noted hearing loss and inability to close her eyes completely during sleep. CPK level was 150 IU/L; EMG demonstrated myopathic motor units in the proximal arm muscles and in both tibialis anterior muscles. Ear, nose, and throat (ENT) evaluation demonstrated sensorimotor deafness. Eye exam showed retinal telangiectasias.

The likely diagnosis is:

1. Davidenkow syndrome
2. Coats syndrome
3. Hopkins syndrome
4. Parsonage Turner syndrome
5. None of the above

DIAGNOSIS

- Coats syndrome is a rare extra-muscular complication of FSHD associated with large D4Z4 contraction.
- High-frequency hearing loss and retinal telangiectasias are required for the diagnosis.
- Uni- or bilateral sensorineural hearing loss is reported in 60% of FSHD patients, and more than 50% of patients have abnormal fluorescein angiography. Retinal vasculopathy may result in retinal detachment. If retinal vasculopathy is detected early, photocoagulation may prevent serious consequences. Annual hearing and ophthalmological examination is recommended.
- Coats syndrome occurs more frequently in female patients with FSHD with large D4Z4 contraction and has a variable age of onset (1–53 years).
- Males tend to develop symptoms earlier and more severely than females. By age 30 years, almost all males and only two-thirds of females exhibit symptoms of FSHD.

CASE 11.5: SCAPULAR WINGING AND BILATERAL FOOT DROP

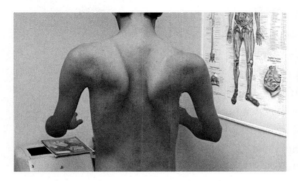

VIDEO 11.5

A 20-year-old Hispanic man presented with a 5-year history of arm weakness and tripping. His examination is demonstrated.

Scapuloperoneal syndrome (SPS) may be caused by all of the following except:

1. FSHD
2. Acid maltase deficiency
3. Myofibrillar myopathy (desminopathy)
4. Duchenne muscular dystrophy (MD)
5. Scapuloperoneal neuronopathy

DIAGNOSIS

- SPS is defined by weakness of the shoulder girdle muscles, leading to bilateral scapular winging, and peroneal muscles, leading to bilateral foot drop.
- Many neuromuscular disorders may present with such a distribution including:
  - Myotonic dystrophy
  - LGMD 2 A
  - Desminopathy
  - Acid maltase deficiency
  - Inclusion body myositis (IBM)
  - Myophosphorylase deficiency
  - Polymyositis
  - Congenital myopathies
  - Nonaka distal myopathy
  - FSHD
  - Hereditary neuropathy with liability to pressure palsy (HNPP)
  - Some cases of spinal muscular atrophy
- Usually, the weakness spreads to other muscles that are characteristically involved in these diseases.
- After exclusion of these diseases, some patients continue to have unclassified scapuloperoneal weakness, and these are classified into two categories:
  1. Scapuloperoneal muscular dystrophy:
     - X-linked dominant SPS (hyalin body myopathy) localized to chromosome Xq. It is caused by mutation of the FAHL1 gene.
     - Autosomal recessive form localized to 3p22
     - CK is slightly elevated and EMG is myopathic. Muscle biopsy is nonspecific but can show hyaline bodies.
  2. Scapuloperoneal neuropathy (Dawidenkow syndrome):
     - Autosomal dominant disease with scapuloperoneal weakness, distal sensory impairment, pes cavus, areflexia, and motor slowing.
     - In some cases, chromosome 17p11.2 deletions are found (a variant of HNPP).
- With genetic advances, this syndrome will yield to more specific genetic categories.
- The workup of SPS includes measurement of CK levels and an EMG to differentiate the myopathic from the neuropathic types. Genetic studies, and possibly a muscle biopsy, are also performed to define the diagnosis and rule out the other mentioned possibilities.

CASE 11.6: SCAPULAR WINGING AND SEVERE SHOULDER PAIN

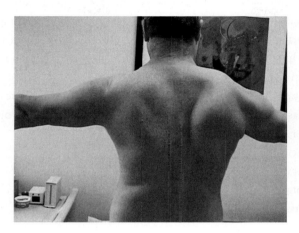

VIDEO 11.6

A 53-year-old man presented with sudden onset severe burning pain of the right shoulder that was preceded by cough and fever 2 weeks earlier. The patient lost the ability to raise his right arm 2 weeks later. EMG demonstrated denervation of the right serratus anterior and deltoid muscles.

The likely diagnosis is:

1. Parsonage Turner syndrome
2. Long thoracic nerve injury
3. C5 cervical radiculopathy
4. Mononeuritis multiplex
5. Guillain-Barré syndrome

DIAGNOSIS

- Examination demonstrated mild atrophy of the right deltoid (suprascapular nerve) and prominent medial winging of the right scapula (serratus anterior, long thoracic nerve).
- Parsonage Turner syndrome, or neuralgic amyotrophy, is due to an acute patchy inflammation of the brachial plexus that may be triggered by a viral upper respiratory infection (URI), immunization, stress, surgery, or childbirth.
- Typically, it starts with severe nocturnal burning pain in the periscapular and shoulder regions that lasts for about 2 weeks, followed by weakness and atrophy of muscles supplied by one or more of the following nerves:
  1. Long thoracic nerve
  2. Axillary nerve
  3. Musculocutaneous nerve
  4. Suprascapular nerve
  5. Phrenic nerve
  6. Anterior interosseous nerve
  7. Spinal accessory nerve
  8. Lingual nerve
- In 30% of cases, the other side is affected simultaneously or within a few weeks.
- EMG shows denervation of the affected muscles.
- Nerve conduction study (NCS) reveals loss of sensory responses of the affected nerves.
- Prognosis is good. Improvement starts a month after the onset, and maximum recovery may take up to 2 years.
- When the long thoracic nerve is affected, scapular winging is the main feature.
  - The winging is medial, meaning that the scapula moves medially when the arms are pushed outstretched against a wall.
  - This is different from the lateral winging due to involvement of dorsal scapular or spinal accessory nerves.
    - Rhomboid weakness is more prominent when the arms are pushed posteriorly against resistance.
    - Trapezius weakness is associated with depressed shoulder and more winging when the arms are abducted.
- It is a self-limiting disease and steroids are not warranted. Judicious pain management is usually needed for severe pain, along with rehabilitation.

CASE 11.7: SUBACUTE SCAPULAR WINGING AND WEAKNESS OF FINGER FLEXORS

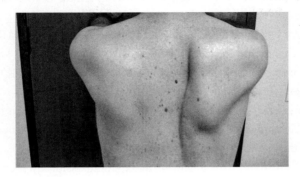

VIDEO 11.7

A 47-year-old man presented with acute unilateral shoulder pain followed by right arm and fingers weakness.

Weakness of the fingers flexion in this case is most likely due to involvement of the following nerve:

1. Long thoracic nerve
2. Anterior interosseous nerve
3. Suprascapular nerve
4. Ulnar nerve
5. Median nerve, main trunk

DIAGNOSIS

- Anterior interosseus neuropathy (AIN) involves a motor branch of the median nerve above the elbow.
- It supplies flexor pollicis longus (FPL), flexor digitorum profundus (FDP) of the 3rd and 4th fingers, and pronator quadratus (PQ).
- Dysfunction of these muscles leads to inability to produce the "OK" sign due to lack of flexion of the terminal phalanges of the first two fingers.
- The affected muscles can be tested electromyographically. Median sensory response is normal because it branches off the median nerve proximal to the lesion.
- AIN is one of the common targets of Parsonage Turner syndrome.
  - Other causes of AIN invovlement include: Compression by pronator teres, bicipital tendon bursa, and trauma.
- Recovery occurs spontaneously in 50% of cases.
- In patients with Martin Gruber anastomosis, atrophy of the intrinsic hands muscles (normally supplied by the ulnar nerve) can be diagnostically confusing.

CASE 11.8: FAMILIAL SCAPULAR WINGING

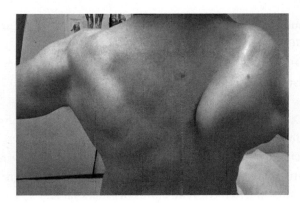

VIDEO 11.8

A 59-year-old man presented with a 10-year history of painless asymmetrical bilateral foot drop. A fraternal twin brother had similar symptoms. CK level was 450 U/L. EMG was myopathic. D4Z4 alleles were normal. Muscle biopsy revealed chronic myopathic changes with several inflammatory foci.

The most appropriate next test is:

1. SMCHD1 gene mutation analysis
2. DMPK gene mutation analysis
3. Dystrophin staining in muscle
4. Calpain gene sequencing
5. Dysferlin western blot analysis

DIAGNOSIS

- FSHD is an autosomal dominant disease. Sporadic mutations occur in 20% of cases of FSHD 1 and 70% of FSHD2 cases.
- 95% of FSHD patients have deletion of D4Z4 gene on chromosome 4. Severity of the disease correlates with size of mutation in FSDH 1 but not in FSHD 2.
- False positives may occur due to non-pathogenic contraction of D4Z4 gene. In atypical cases of FSHD, the pathogenicity of D4Z4 mutations should be confirmed by looking for a permissive distal sequence (4qA).
- In 5% of FSHD cases, there is no contraction in D4Z4 gene, yet they maintain an opening of the chromatin structure at the D4Z4 locus. These cases are designated FSHD 2.
  - FSHD2 requires inheritance of two unlinked genetic factors: 1) a permissive 4qA allele and 2) a loss of function mutation of the *SMCHD1* gene which is found on chromosome 18p11.
  - FSHD 2 presents similarly to FSHD 1. Onset age is usually older (more than 30 years).
  - Patients with severe weakness may have both FSDH 1 and FSHD 2 mutations.
  - Facial sparing, as in this case, occurs in 15% of cases and is usually associated with smaller deletions.
  - Muscle inflammation, as in this case, occurs in 75% of cases.

REFERENCE

Digenic inheritance of an SMCHD1 mutation and an FSHD-permissive D4Z4 allele causes facioscapulo-humeral muscular dystrophy type 2. *Nature Genet.* 2012;44:1370–1374.

CASE 11.9: SCAPULAR WINGING AND A CK OF 2,000 IU/L

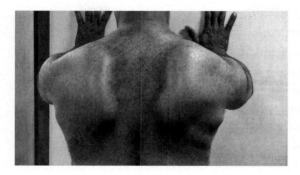

VIDEO 11.9

A 57-year-old man presented with a 5-year history of difficulty walking. Two years later, he could not lift his arms. Examination also showed elbows contractures and hearing loss. He had normal sural responses and myopathic EMG. CK was 2,000 U/L. Chest X-ray revealed cardiomegaly. Muscle biopsy showed chronic myopathic changes. There was no neurogenic atrophy or evidence of metabolic or mitochondrial myopathy. He did not know much about his parent's history.

Testing for which of the following is most appropriate?

1. Acid maltase activity in a dry blood spot
2. FHL1 mutation
3. FSHD 2 gene mutation
4. HNPP mutation
5. Calpain muscle tissue staining

DIAGNOSIS

- Among the mentioned findings, the presence of contractures, cardiomegaly, and hearing loss suggested scapuloperoneal myopathy due to FHL1 gene mutation.
- Four and a half LIM protein 1 (FHL 1) mutation is the cause of four different phenotypes:
  - Reducing body myopathy
  - Emery Dreifuss muscular dystrophy
  - X-linked myopathy characterized by postural muscle atrophy
  - Scapuloperoneal myopathy (SPM)
    - It is an X-linked dominant disease
    - Usual age of onset is late twenties
    - Slowly progressive distal leg (foot drop) and proximal arm weakness
    - Males are more severely affected than females and at an earlier age, and most of them become wheelchair bound
    - Scapular winging
    - Late onset joints contractures
    - Cardiomyopathy is a common cause of death
    - Respiratory involvement is not common
    - CK: 2–10 times normal
    - Reducing bodies are seen in the muscle biopsy
    - The pathogenic mechanism by which FHL1 mutations cause human muscle disease is not clear. Despite heterogeneous phenotypes, a common pathogenic mechanism is suggested.

REFERENCE

Wilding BR, et al. FHL1 mutations that cause clinically distinct human myopathies form protein aggregates and impair myoblast differentation. *J Cell Sci.* 2014;Mar 14.

PROXIMAL ARM WEAKNESS

DIAGNOSIS

- LEMS does not usually respond well to any of the mentioned modalities. Most patients require substantial and prolonged use of immunosuppressive therapy for modest improvement of symptoms.
- Clinical severity does not correlate with the level of voltage gated calcium channel antibodies.
- In order to increase the acetylcholine available at the postsynaptic membrane, one will have to:
  - Reverse the pathological attack against the calcium channels in the presynaptic membrane (immunomodulatory therapy) or
  - Interfere with the acetylcholine release mechanism (symptomatic therapy)
  - Decreased acetylcholine degradation by choline esterase
- 3,4 DAP prolongs depolarization of the presynaptic membrane and thereby increases calcium entry to the presynaptic terminal and results in release of ACh.
  - It improves both motor and autonomic dysfunction.
  - 20mg QID is the max dose.
  - It is not FDA approved but can be obtained from compounding pharmacies.
- Acetylcholinesterase inhibitors reduce the metabolism of acetylcholine and thereby increase the amount available at the binding sites. Alone, they have a marginal effect. They are commonly used along with 3,4 DAP.
- Immunologic therapies:
  - Reserved for severe symptoms that do not respond to 3,4 DAP.
  - Prednisone, azathioprine, IVIG, PLEX, and rituximab are all reported to be effective to some extent.
- Cases of LEMS that are not associated with malignancies have a better survival rate.
- Treatment of the underlying malignancy may lead to remission of LEMS. Unfortunately, most associated cancers are not curable.

REFERENCE

Maddison P, et al. Long term outcome in Lambert-Eaton myasthenic syndrome without cancer. *J Neurol Neurosurg Psychiatry.* 2001;70:212–217.

CASE 12.6: CHRONIC PROXIMAL ARM WEAKNESS

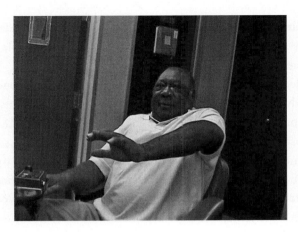

VIDEO 12.6

A 60-year-old man presented with a 15-year history of difficulty climbing stairs and lifting arms. Symptoms gradually progressed. He had no distal weakness, reflexes abnormalities, dysphagia, or abnormal sensory findings. He had three healthy daughters. CK level was 2,200–3,300 U/L. EMG revealed many short duration and polyphasic units in the proximal arm and leg muscles. There were no spontaneous discharges. Muscle biopsy showed remarkable variation of fiber size and shape, many internal nuclei, split fibers, and rare necrotic fibers. There was no inflammation. Dystrophic proteins immunohistochemistry and western blot analyses were negative including Dystrophin, sarcoglycans, dysferlin, calpain, and caveoline.

This case is classified as:

1. Polymyositis
2. Becker muscular dystrophy
3. Myotonic dystrophy
4. Limb girdle muscular dystrophy (LGMD), undetermined type
5. Facioscapulohumeral muscular dystrophy (FSHD)

DIAGNOSIS

- Limb girdle muscular dystrophy is a descriptive term that was popular when muscle diseases were classified according to the distribution of weakness (Table 12.6.1).
- LGMD became a "wastebasket" for all non-classified myopathies.
  - In the last decade, most of the contents of the "basket" became genetically oriented.
  - Molecular advances identified the muscle cell membrane's components and their functions.
  - Deficiency of different proteins lead to different types of LGMD and the genes that code for most of these proteins have been identified.
  - While treatment of LGMD has not significantly changed in the last 50 years, the molecular and genetic basis of many of these disorders has become clear, and hopefully this is a step toward a curative approaches through genetic engineering and stem cell transplantation.
- Genetic advances have limited the utility of muscle biopsy in the diagnosis of most of these disorders. If the phenotype suggests a specific type of LGMD, then a blood sample may be adequate for the diagnosis.
- Even the most exhaustive investigations leave 30% of LGMD unclassified.
- Even when a specific form of LGMD is suspected, many insurance companies deny payment because such a diagnosis does not change management. The impact of a specific diagnosis on the prognosis and genetic counseling should be emphasized to facilitate insurance payment.
- The exact defect in the presented case was not identified. The frozen muscle tissue along with others is awaiting a new round of studies based on the newly identified defects or a research protocol.

TABLE 12.6.1 Classification of limb girdle dystrophies (LGMDs)

- Autosomal dominant:
  - LGMD 1A AD 5q22.3–31.3 Myotilin
  - LGMD 1B AD 1q11–21 Lamin A/C
  - LGMD 1C AD 3p25 Caveolin-3
  - LGMD 1D AD 6q23?
  - LGMD 1E AD 7q?
  - LGMD 1F AD 7q31.1–32.2
- Autosomal recessive:
  - LGMD 2A AR 15q15.1–21.1 Calpain-3
  - LGMD 2B* AR 2p13 Dysferlin
  - LGMD 2C AR 13q12 -Sarcoglycan
  - LGMD 2D AR 17q12–21.3 -Sarcoglycan
  - LGMD 2E AR 4q12 -Sarcoglycan
  - LGMD 2F AR 5q33–34 -Sarcoglycan
  - LGMD 2G AR 17q11–12 Telethonin
  - LGMD 2H** AR 9q31–33 E3-ubiquitin-ligase (TRIM 32)
  - LGMD 2I AR 19q13 Fukutin-related protein (FKRP)
  - LGMD 2J AR 2q31 Titin
  - LGMD 2K AR 9q31 POMT1
  - LGMD 2L AR 9q31–33 Fukutin
  - LGMD 2M AR 1p32 POMGnT1

REFERENCE

Amato A, Russell J. *Neuromuscular disorders*. New York: Mc Graw Hill; 2008.

CASE 12.7: PROXIMAL ARM WEAKNESS AND CARDIOMYOPATHY

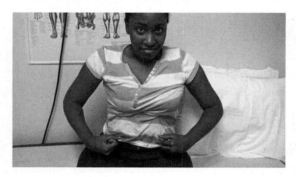

VIDEO 12.7

A 25-year-old woman presented with symptoms starting at age 10 years and consisted of difficulty arising from chairs and lifting her arms to do her hair. Progressively, she became weaker and she developed bilateral foot drop and mild quadriceps weakness. She developed orthopnea. Echocardiogram revealed an ejection fraction of 30%. EMG revealed many short duration polyphasic units in the proximal and distal muscles of the arms and legs and no spontaneous discharges in the thoracic paraspinal muscles. CPK level was 1,840–2,300 U/L repeatedly. Muscle biopsy showed end stage muscle disease with few fibers with rimmed vacuoles.

In this case of LGMD, the following features suggest Telethonin mutation:

1. Cardiomyopathy
2. Quads weakness
3. CK level
4. Vacuoles in the muscle biopsy
5. All of the above

DIAGNOSIS

- Telethonin is localized to skeletal and cardiac muscles, and it is a substrate of serine kinase domain of titin.
- Age of onset is 9–15 years.
- Weakness affects proximal and distal leg muscles (quadriceps and tibialis anterior) and proximal arm muscles. Facial and neck muscles are usually saved.
- Patients progresses to non-ambulatory state in the 3rd or 4th decade of life in 40% of cases.
- Cardiomyopathy occurs in 50% of cases.
- CK level is increased 3- to 30-fold.
- Muscle pathology usually shows dystrophic myopathy, lobulated fibers, rimmed vacuoles, and absent telethonin staining.

CASE 12.8: PROXIMAL WEAKNESS AND HARD BREASTS

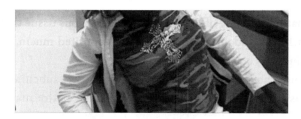

VIDEO 12.8

A 50-year-old woman with chronic renal failure has been on hemodialysis for 5 years. She had multiple gadolinium enhanced MRIs for chronic lower back pain (LBP). She became unable to raise her arms and legs, which evolved over 6 months. She had no dysphagia. She was found to have hard skin and breasts, and her CK level and EMG were normal.

The most likely diagnosis is:

1. Scleroderma
2. Polymyositis
3. Nephrogenic systemic sclerosis (NSS)
4. Polymyalgia rheumatica
5. Systemic calcinosis

DIAGNOSIS

- The diffuse loss of reflexes and severe proximal weakness and motor slowing with conduction block and elevated CSF protein suggested an inflammatory demyelinating neuropathy. The temporal profile of the first episode suggested GBS as there was no more progression after 4 weeks of the onset.
- Recurrence of the disease a few months later indicated that the first episode was most likely part of relapsing remitting CIDP. About 2%–4% of patients who are diagnosed initially with GBS turn out to have CIDP as the future course unfolds.
- Distinguishing acute onset CIDP from fluctuating GBS is difficult but important because steroids are contraindicated in GBS and maintenance treatment is often needed in CIDP. The prognosis and associated diseases are not the same.
- If worsening occurs within 8 weeks of the onset of symptoms, differentiation is not that easy. CIDP is usually the diagnosis if the disease relapses after 8 weeks of the first episode.
- Features that favor the diagnosis of GBS are facial involvement and dysautonomia. The presence of significant distal sensory impairment and loss of sural responses is more in favor of CIDP.

REFERENCE

Ruts L, Drenthen J, Jacobs BC, van Doorn PA; Dutch GBS Study Group. Distinguishing acute-onset CIDP from fluctuating Guillain-Barre syndrome: a prospective study. *Neurology.* 2010 May 25;74(21):1680–1686. doi:10.1212/WNL.0b013e3181e07d14. Epub 2010 Apr 28.

CASE 12.10: PROGRESSIVE PROXIMAL WEAKNESS AND CARDIOMYOPATHY

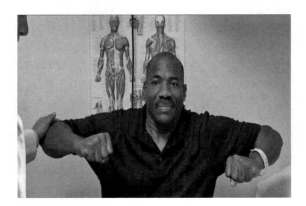

VIDEO 12.10

A 54-year-old-man presented with progressive shortness of breath of a few months duration. His ejection fraction was 20% and coronary arteriogram was normal. CK level was 3,400 U/L. Myocardiac biopsy revealed endomysial inflammation. Left ventricular assist device was inserted. No cause was found for the increased CK level. After several admissions to the hospital, he was found to have proximal weakness. Glucosidase acid alpha dry blood spot was negative. Muscle biopsy (Figures 12.10.1 and 12.10.2) showed inflammatory myopathy. Extremities strength normalized with steroids but not the congestive cardiac failure (CCF). He was placed on cardiac transplantation list.

Which of the following is true about cardiac/pulmonary involvement in myopathy?

1. Cardiomyopathy can be the presenting feature of polymyositis (PM).
2. Cardiomyopathy and inflammatory myopathy can be explained by dystrophinopathy.
3. Dyspnea out of proportion to muscle weakness is seen in acid maltase deficiency.
4. His muscle weakness was all due to CCF.
5. Cardiac involvement associated with polymyositis is usually responsive to treatment of PM.

DIAGNOSIS

- PLEX is shown in multiple studies to be as effective as IVIG for the treatment of CIDP.
- 80% of virgin CIDP cases respond to PLEX, but 66% of them relapse within 2 weeks of discontinuation. All improved with subsequent interval PLEX therapy. Long-term immunosupression with azathioprine or similar agents may be needed to reduce the reliability on PLEX.
- IVIG is used as the first line due to the perceived high risk of complications of PLEX and more availability of IVIG. Fifty percent of IVIG refractory cases respond to PLEX.
- However, with the availability of smaller and well-computerized PLEX machines that can be made available on an outpatient basis, PLEX can be given the same consideration as the IVIG. Complication rate is comparable to IVIG and is mostly related to venous access.
- The best outcome measure in CIDP is proximal weakness. Sensory ataxia, distal weakness, and deep tendon reflexes (DTRs) are the last to improve.
- Patients that may benefit from PLEX more than IVIG include ones with:
  - Congestive cardiac failure: fluid volume can be adjusted to negative during PLEX, but fluid overload can easily be precipitated by IVIG.
  - Renal impairment, especially in diabetics: IVIG may worsen renal function but PLEX does not.
  - Recurrent DVT
  - In CIDP cases, IgG monoclonal gammopathy is more responsive to PLEX than IgM monoclonal gammopathy.

REFERENCE

Hahn CF, et al. Plasma-exchange therapy in chronic inflammatory demyelinating polyneuropathy: a double blind, sham-controlled, crossover study. *Brain.* 1996;119:1055–1066.

CASE 13.4: ACUTE MYALGIA AND ELEVATED CK LEVEL

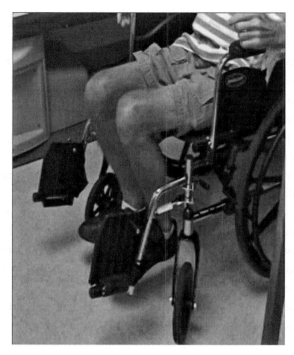

VIDEO 13.4

A 65-year-old man had subacute myalgia and progressive proximal weakness in the arms and legs. Creatine Kinase (CK) level was 7,500 U/L. EMG: see Video 13.4. Muscle biopsy showed severe muscle necrosis with no inflammation, SRP antibodies were positive. Response to steroids was poor.

The most likely diagnosis is:

1. Polymyositis (PM)
2. Vasculitis
3. Necrotizing myopathy (NM)
4. Inclusion body myositis (IBM)
5. Viral myositis

DIAGNOSIS

- Becker muscular dystrophy (BMD) should be considered in the differential diagnoses of several presentations in male adults, including limb girdle weakness, isolated quadriceps weakness, asymptomatic hyperCKemia, muscle cramps, rhabdomyolysis, and cardio-myopathy. The diagnosis is not difficult when all these abnormalities exist in the same patients, but they may be present individually, and in these cases, the diagnosis is usually delayed.
- The lack of family history is not exclusive as 10% of cases are due to spontaneous mutations.
- Calves pseudohypertophy is a useful sign.
- The most common presentation is walking difficulty after age 15 years. Fifty percent of patients lose the ability to walk by age 40.
- CK elevation is usually 20–200 times normal. EMG is myopathic in the affected muscles.
- MRI has become a popular tool in the neuromuscular clinic in the last decade. It was used in this case to demonstrate the fatty replacement of calf muscles.
- Muscle biopsy shows dystrophic myopathy. Dystrophin is decreased uniformly or in a patchy pattern, unlike Duchenne muscular dystrophy (DMD), where it is absent. WB analysis typically reveals decreased amount or size of dystrophin.
- There is a 50% chance that the daughters of this male will be carriers. Carriers are usually asymptomatic but they may display mild weakness or muscle pain. The more sensitive way to diagnose carriers is WB analysis and not CK or muscle biopsy.
- While steroids are commonly used to treat Duchenne muscular dystrophy (DMD) patients, they are not recommended in BMD except in very progressive cases.
- There is no promising treatment modality in the horizon. Genetic engineering and stem cell transplantation may provide a glimpse of hope to the future.
- Annual ECG is recommended to detect conduction abnormalities early.

CASE 13.8: DYSTROPHIC MYOPATHY WITH INFLAMMATION

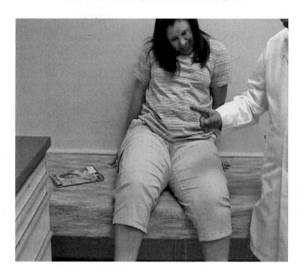

VIDEO 13.8

A 32-year-old woman had a 7-year history of difficulty climbing stairs followed by weakness of the hand grips and frequent falls. CK levels were 3,000–9,000 U/L and EMG revealed myopathy with thoracic paraspinal fibrillations. Muscle biopsy revealed chronic myopathy with lymphocytic inflammatory changes. She did not respond to 6 months of IVIG treatment and 1 year of treatment with methotrexate. There is no family history. Our neuromuscular exam revealed the following medical research council (MRC) power grades: hip flexion: 0, knee extension: 3, knee flexion: 3, ankle extension: 2, ankle flexion: 3, wrist extension: 4, fingers flexion: 3, neck flexion: 4, neck extension: 5. There was no facial weakness or scapular winging.

These findings are consistent with:

1. Dysferlinopathy
2. Dystrophinopathy
3. Calpainopathy
4. Caveolinopathy
5. Myotilinopathy

DIAGNOSIS

- Imaging of the thoracic spinal cord is often missed in evaluation of patients with sensory ataxia and hyperreflexia due to the infrequent involvement of the thoracic cord with spondylotic myelopathy compared to the cervical cord. However, lesions such as herniated disc, meningeoma, metastatic tumors, and lymphoma are important causes of thoracic myelopathy.

- After exclusion of compression myelopathies, investigations should be directed to non-compressive causes such as B_{12} deficiency, copper deficiency, adrenal myeloneuropathy, hereditary spastic paraplegia (HSP), tropical spastic paraplegia, HIV vacuolar myelopathy, and so on.

- The confinement of the symptoms and signs to the legs raised the possibility of thoracic myelopathy despite the lack of a clear sensory level. Thoracic spine MRI did reveal T5 cord compression by a large herniated disk.

- Commonly, an MRI of the lumbosacral area is ordered to look for an explanation of sensory and motor symptoms restricted to the legs with hyperreflexia. However, the spinal cord ends at L1 level, and pathology below that level would not explain the hyperreflexia and ataxia.

CASE 13.11: PROXIMAL WEAKNESS AFTER BONE MARROW TRANSPLANTATION

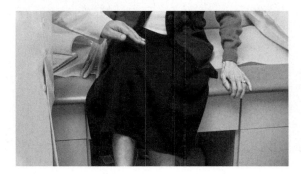

VIDEO 13.11

A 56-year-old woman had a history of allogenic bone marrow transplantation for myelofibrosis 2.5 years earlier with previous use of tacrolimus. She presented with subacute myalgia, weakness, fever, and skin induration. Examination: induration of skin, moderate proximal weakness and normal sensation. CPK level was 1,200 U/L. EMG revealed irritative myopathy. Muscle biopsy is shown in Figures 13.11.1 and 13.11.2.

The following should be considered in the differential diagnosis:

1. Idiopathic polymyositis
2. Graft versus host disease (GVHD) associated PM
3. Tacrolimus induced polymyositis
4. Dermatomyositis
5. Inclusion body myositis (IBM)

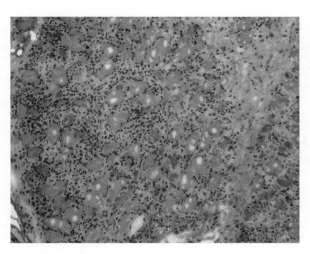

FIGURE 13.11.1 Severe endomysial inflammation.

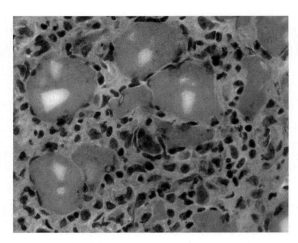

FIGURE 13.11.2 Severe endomysial inflammation.

DIAGNOSIS

- Graft versus host disease (GVHD) is a major complication of bone marrow transplantation and it can mimic autoimmune disease like scleroderma, dermatomyositis, polymyositis, medication-induced myositis, and sicca syndrome.
- GVHD develops in 33%–64% of allogenic stem cells transplantation (SCT) and is more common with advancing age and in patients with a history of acute GVHD.
- It is a multiorgan disease that can develop months to years after the graft.
- Involvement of skeletal muscles is rare (less than 1% of patients who undergo bone marrow transplantation) and even more rare when skeletal muscles are the main target. The incidence of myositis is not related to the underlying disease that was treated with bone marrow transplantation.
- A study has shown that GVHD-induced myositis developed anywhere between 7 and 55 months after transplantation.
- CK ranged between 454 and 8,400 U/L.
- EMG: irritative myopathy.
- Muscle biopsy showed inflammatory myopathy in 80% of cases.
- All patients have involvement of other organs, mostly skin and liver. The skin lesions are different from those of dermatomyositis. The skin is diffusely indurated and firm with mild erythema.
- They respond well to steroids and azathioprine or cyclosporine.
- Tacrolimus is reported to cause polymyositis, but no skin lesions are reported. Yet, it may be better to replace it with another immunosuppressive agent in this case.
- Pathological identification of the type of cells in the muscle lesions can determine if the cells are donor related, thus confirming GVHD.

REFERENCES

Stevens AM, Sullivan KM, Nelson JL. Polymyositis as a manifestation of chronic graft-versus-host disease. *Rheumatology*. 2003;42:34–39.

Allen JA, Greenberg SA, Amato AA. Dermatomyositis-like muscle pathology in patients with chronic graft-versus-host disease. *Muscle Nerve*. 2009;40:643–647.

CHAPTER 14

QUADRICEPS WEAKNESS

CASE 14.1: SEVERE THIGH PAIN AND WEAKNESS

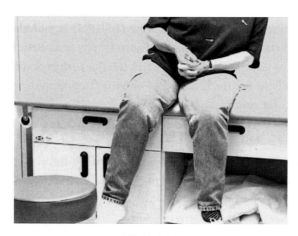

VIDEO 14.1

A 43-year-old non-diabetic woman had woken up with severe left thigh burning pain that mandated an ER visit. The pain was barely responsive to hydrocodone every 4 hours. Two weeks later she started losing her balance. A few weeks later she had weakness of the right leg. Examination is shown. She also had absent knee jerks. Lumbar spines magnetic resonance imaging (LS MRI) was not remarkable. HbA1c was 5.5%. Electromyogram (EMG) showed active denervation of the bilateral anterior and medial thigh muscles and glutei. Lumbosarcal (LS) paraspinal muscles also showed fibrillations and positive sharp waves. Nerve conduction study (NCS) revealed a mild sensory neuropathy.

The features suggest:

1. Non-diabetic LS radiculoplexus neuropathy (LSRPN)
2. Compressive LS polyradiculopathy
3. Diabetic polyneuropathy
4. Herpes Zoster radiculitis
5. Paraneoplastic syndrome

DIAGNOSIS

- The typical case of IBM presents with several years' history of loss of balance and falls due to quadriceps weakness, and it usually affects white males after age 50 years.
- Simultaneously, there is weakness of the finger flexors and sometimes bilateral foot drop.
- A typical pattern of weakness affects quadriceps more than iliopsoas, and biceps more than deltoids.
- Facial weakness occurs in 30% of cases, and dysphagia occurs in the majority of cases at one point, though it can be the presenting feature.
- CK is usually mildly elevated and EMG shows mixed short- and long-duration potentials indicating chronicity.
- Muscle biopsy usually shows chronic myopathic findings with eosinophilic cytoplasmic inclusions, red-rimmed vacuoles, congophilia, and endomysial inflammation in variable proportions and to variable degrees.
- The following atypical features are not uncommon, at least at the time of presentation, but eventually most of the diagnostic criteria are met:
  1. Polymyositis-like phenotype
  2. Isolated quadriceps weakness
  3. Isolated finger flexor weakness
  4. Severe dysphagia at presentation
  5. CK higher than 10 times normal
  6. Polymyositis-like pathology (leading to misdiagnosis of PM)
- It seems that the initial inflammatory phase is associated with high CK level and severe endomysial inflammation, but a few years later, a degenerative phase supervenes and is characterized by mild CK elevation and the presence of vacuoles and inclusions in the biopsy.
- The most common cause of refractory "polymyositis" is IBM.
- No clinical trial demonstrated efficacy of steroids, IVIG, chemotherapeutic agents, or interferon in IBM.

CASE 14.4: BIG BUT WEAK CALVES

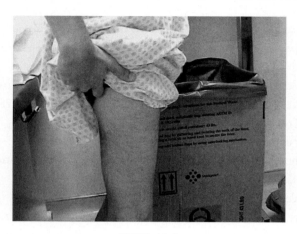

VIDEO 14.4

A 26-year-old man presented with gradually evolving difficulty climbing stairs. Examination is shown. CPK level was 5,000 U/L. EMG revealed many short duration polyphasic units in the proximal and distal arm and leg muscles. None of his three brothers was affected.

Calves hypertrophy is a feature of:

1. Becker muscular dystrophy
2. Amyloid myopathy
3. Charcot-Marie-Tooth disease (CMT) Type 1A
4. Fukayama congenital muscular dystrophy (CMD)
5. Neuromyotonia

DIAGNOSIS

Hypertrophy of the calves is commonly seen in neuromuscular clinics.

It is clinically useful to differentiate between several types of calves hypertrophy:

- Hypertrophy due to replacement of muscle by other tissue (pseudohypertrophy). Depending on the type of tissue the following subtypes are recognized:
  - ◆ Fatty tissue replacement such as in dystrophinopathies
  - ◆ Amyloid structure replacement such as in systemic amyloidosis
  - ◆ Glycosaminoglycans such as in hypothyroidism. In this condition there is also an increase in the endomysial connective tissue.
  - ◆ D-glycogen deposition: debrancher enzyme deficiency
- Reinnervation: chronic denervating conditions usually are associated with significant reinnervation and sometimes hypertrophy such as CMT and S1 radiculopathy.
- Due to hyperactivity of muscle fibers such as in neuromyotonia
- Myotonic disorders such as myotonia congenita
- Sarcoglycanopathy (LGMD 2C-F), telethoninopathy (LGMD 2G), and LGMD 2I (FKRP)
- Focal enlargement: neoplasm, inflammation

Muscle sonography provides an objective measurement of calf girths and can determine the type of hypertrophy. Calves hypertrophy and thighs weakness is typically seen in dystrophinopathies.

REFERENCES

Reimers CD, et al. Calf enlargement in neuromuscular diseases: a quantitative ultrasound study in 350 patients and review of the literature. *J Neurol Sci*. 1996 Nov;143(1–2):46–56.

Praveen K, et al. HoffMann's syndrome: a rare neurological presentation of hypothyroidism. *Int J Nutr Pharmacol Neurol Dis*. 2011;1:201–203.

CASE 14.5: PROGRESSIVE WEAKNESS AND DIFFUSE DENERVATION

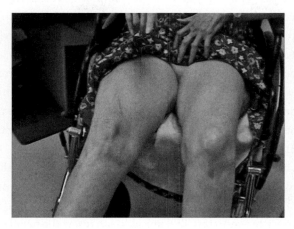

VIDEO 14.5

A 70-Year-old woman presented with a 6-month history of difficulty walking and falls. She became wheelchair bound. Examination revealed weakness and atrophy of the anterior thighs and forelegs and mild proximal arm weakness. Sensation was normal. Deep tendon reflexes were 3+ in the legs and arms. CK level was 340 U/L. MRI of the entire spine was normal. EMG revealed fibrillations and positive sharp waves in the proximal and distal leg muscles bilaterally and thoracic paraspinal muscles and few fibrillations in the proximal arm muscles.

The most likely cause of thigh weakness in this case is:

1. Limb girdle muscular dystrophy (LGMD)
2. Amyotrophic lateral sclerosis (ALS)
3. Becker muscular dystrophy
4. Diabetic amyotrophy
5. LS radiculopathy

DIAGNOSIS

- Thoracic paraspinal (TPS) muscles have a very important role in the neuromuscular diagnostic process due to the facts that:
  - They are rarely affected by spondylosis that usually affects the cervical and lumbosacral spines due to their curvatures and weight-bearing properties.
  - The are affected early in denervating conditions due to their proximity to the motor neurons to which they are connected by short posterior spinal rami.
- TPS muscles involvement in ALS provides an affected segment to the three out of four required segments (cranial, cervical, thoracic, and lumbosacral) for the diagnosis of ALS according to El Escorial criteria.
- TPS muscles are also affected early in inflammatory and metabolic myopathies as they show evidence of increased irritability in a form of fibrillations and positive sharp waves.
- The most appropriate way to test TPS muscles is to insert the needle right adjacent to the corresponding spinous process until a resistance is met due to the transverse processes; then the needle is pulled a few millimeters.
- It is important to remember that the myotome level does not correspond to the spine levels due to the fact that the spinal cord is shorter that the spinal column.
- Poor relaxation is the most important hurdle in the way of examination of the TPS muscle. This can be minimized by optimizing room temperature, explaining the procedure to the patient, and positioning the patient on the side and flexing the hips and head.
- In the presented case, the progressive course, atrophy, hyperreflexia, normal sensation, and diffuse denervation argued for ALS.

CASE 14.6: PROGRESSIVE CALVES ATROPHY AND ELEVATED CK

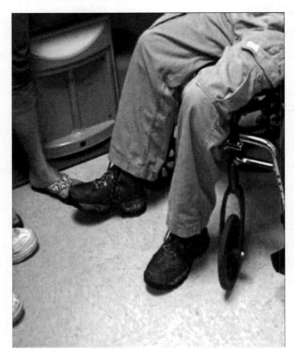

VIDEO 14.6

A 27-year-old-man noticed 10 years earlier an inability to stand on toes. He did not seek medical advice. Two years later, he had difficulty climbing stairs. He moved his apartment to the ground floor. Two years later, he could not arise from a chair without help. His exam revealed atrophy of the calves and proximal weakness. CPK level was 4,350 U/L. EMG revealed 40% short duration units in the proximal and distal leg muscles and 2+ fibrillations and positive sharp waves in the TPS muscles.

The most appropriate next test is:

1. Blood sample for dysferlin mutations
2. Muscle biopsy for dysferlin staining
3. Blood sample for calpain mutations
4. Muscle biopsy for calpain staining
5. Dry blood spot for acid alpha glucosidase activity

DIAGNOSIS

- Dysferlin gene mutation accounts for 1% of unclassified LGMD and 60% of distal myopathies.
- It is allelic to LGMD 2B.
- Western blot (WB) analysis on white blood cells correlates well with WB on muscle tissue.
- On muscle biopsy, absent dysferlin is more significant than patchy staining for accurate diagnosis.
- Patients with absent dysferlin also show abnormal calpain staining, and caution should be taken to avoid erroneous diagnosis of calpainopathy.
- Endomysial inflammation is common in muscle biopsies, leading to erroneous diagnosis of polymyositis.
- Dysferlinopathy may also present as LGMD or even as asymptomatic rhabdomyolysis. Rarely it presents with bilateral foot drop.
- Asymmetry is very usual in Miyoshi myopathy, and that can be a source of confusion with S1 radiculopathy.
- No cardiac involvement is expected in MM.

CASE 14.7: DANCING DIFFICULTY

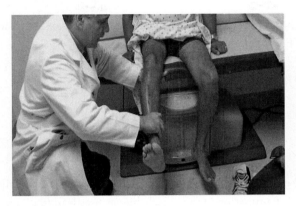

VIDEO 14.7

A 41-year-old man presented with a 10-year history of difficulty holding up his arms and dancing.

The quadriceps atrophy in this case is likely due to:

1. Becker MD
2. Inclusion body myositis
3. Facioscapulohumeral muscular dystrophy (FSHD)
4. Diabetic amyotrophy
5. Scapuloperoneal syndrome

DIAGNOSIS

The demonstrated clinical findings are typically seen in FSHD, except quadriceps weakness. Atypical features of FSHD:

1. Quadriceps weakness
2. Respiratory involvement occurs in 1% of cases
3. Extraocular muscles weakness

Typical features:

1. Asymmetry can be so striking that facial nerve palsy is erroneously diagnosed.
2. Endomysial inflammation in the muscle biopsy may lead to diagnostic confusion with polymyositis.
3. Hearing loss and retinal telangiectasia occur in two-thirds of cases.
4. Distal weakness is common leading to asymmetrical foot drop and weakness of wrist extensors. Hypertrophy of the extensor digitorum brevis (EDB) indicates myopathic rather than neurogenic foot drop.

Quadriceps: selective weakness:

- Hereditary myopathies:
  - Becker muscular dystrophy (BMD)
  - Lim Girdle muscular dystrophy (LGMD): 1B; 2B; 2H; 2L
  - Emery-Dreifuss muscular dystrophy: Lamin A and C
  - Hereditary inclusion body myopathy 3 (HIBM3)
- Inflammatory myopathies:
  - Inclusion body myositis (IBM)
  - Polymyositis with mitochondrial pathology
  - Focal myositis
- Myopathy with ring fibers
- Nerve disorders:
  - Spinal muscular atrophy
    - 5q: Type III & IV
    - Lower extremity dominant
  - Femoral neuropathy
  - Diabetic amyotrophy
  - L3-L4 radiculopathy
  - Lumbo-sacral plexopathies: especially neoplastic

REFERENCE

Tawil R. Facioscapulohumeral muscular dystrophy. *Neurotherapeutics*. 2008 Oct;5(4):601–606.

CASE 14.8A: LEG WEAKNESS AND AREFLEXIA

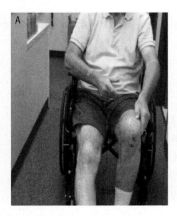

VIDEO 14.8A

A 55-year-old man presented with a 6-month history of progressive gait instability and feet numbness. In addition to what is shown, he had diffuse areflexia. CSF protein was 160mg/dl. IFPE revealed IgM spike. He had severe motor slowing and prolonged distal latencies. He responded to IVIG. Few months later he had a flue like illness followed by severe weakness (shown in the video). His Sulfatide antibody titer was 1:100,000.

The deterioration was likely:

1. An exacerbation of CIDP
2. Due to appearance of Sulfatide antibodies
3. Triggered by a viral illness
4. Due to an unrelated disease
5. Due to monoclonal gammopathy

DIAGNOSIS

- The case meets inflammatory neuropathy cause and treatment (INCAT) diagnostic criteria of CIDP.
- 80% of CIDP cases respond to initial therapy but less than 30% achieve remission off medication.
- Natural course of CIDP:
  - Chronic monophasic: 15%
  - Chronic relapsing-remitting: 34%
  - Stepwise progressive: 15%
  - Steady progressive: 15%
- Monoclonal gammopathy is present in 25% of cases.
  - Unlike GBS, only small number have autoantibodies against myelin protein. IgM is more likely to be pathogenic than IgG and immunofixation protein electrophoresis (IFPE) needs to be monitored for malignant transformation.
- IVIG and PLEX are equally effective in CIDP.
- IVIG has become the treatment of choice, mostly due to convenience and low side effects profile.
- After induction with 2g/kg/bw divided over two days, booster doses and frequency will need to be individualized according to the clinical response and side effects. We use 1gm/kg/bw every month times three, and then reduce the dose and frequency, if tolerated, until completely off. Some cases like the one in this case need more frequent infusions.
- Exacerbations of CIDP are usually triggered by viral infection, emotional stress, surgery, trauma, and vaccination, but frequently, no clear precipitating factors are found.
- The significance of sulfatide antibodies that appear in a minority of CIDP cases is controversial. These cases are difficult to differentiate from regular CIDP cases. They may have more sensory ataxia and tremor and may be less responsive to IVIG.

Therefore, the presence of these antibodies should not affect the way these cases are treated and should not warrant splitting these cases from CIDP.

REFERENCE

Querol L, et al. Long-term outcome in chronic inflammatory demyelinating polyneuropathy patients treated with intravenous immunoglobulin: A retrospective study. *Muscle Nerve*. 2013 Dec;48(6):870–876.

CASE 14.8B: IMPROVED BUT DEVELOPED SWOLLEN LEGS AFTER IVIG

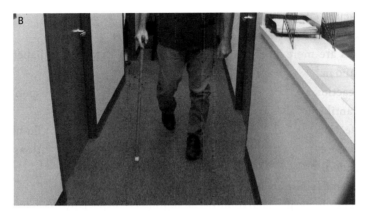

VIDEO 14.8B

The patient responded again to IVIG but could not tolerate less frequency of infusions than weekly. A few months later he developed deep venous thrombosis (DVT).

Complications of IVIG include:

1. DVT
2. Renal impairment
3. Skin rash
4. Aseptic meningitis
5. Flu-like reaction

DIAGNOSIS

- The anterior interosseus nerve is a pure motor nerve that branches off median nerve proximally in the forearm and supplies FDP I, II, FPL, and PQ.
- It can be affected by multiple factors, the most common of which is idiopathic brachial plexitis (Parsonage Turner syndrome). As a matter of fact, it can be the only feature of brachial plexitis.
- No sensory symptoms are expected, but deep forearm pain is common, which can be very severe and may last days or weeks.
- Characteristically, patients cannot pinch or form the letter "O" with their thumb and index finger as there is weakness of flexion of the distal phalanges of these fingers, which are flexed by FDP and FPL (flexor digitorum superficialis, which supplies the middle interphalangeal joint, is supplied by the median nerve before the branching of the anterior interosseous nerve (AIN).
- When AIN is affected, along with other nerves such as the long thoracic nerve, spinal accessory nerve, and suprascapular nerve, the diagnosis of Parsonage Turner syndrome is not hard to make, but when it is the only feature, other causes should be considered, and an attempt to explore and look for a compression is reasonable after 6 months of conservative treatment.
- Other causes include:
  - Fibrous band within pronator teres
  - Compartmental syndrome
  - Soft tissue and PN tumors
  - Ischemia from arteriovenous fistula, or vasculitis
  - Multifocal motor neuropathy
  - Trauma
- The presence of sensory symptoms in the fingers should suggest a more proximal median neuropathy, which has a different set of causes.

CASE 15.2: HAND AND FINGER FLEXOR WEAKNESS AND MYOPATHIC EMG

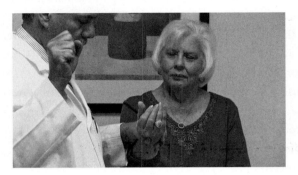

VIDEO 15.2

A 65-year-old woman presented with a 15-year history of slowly progressive weakness of the arms and legs, as demonstrated in the video. She had normal quadriceps strength and no dysphagia. Creatine Kinase (CK) level was normal and EMG revealed mixed long and short duration potentials in the bilateral distal arm and leg muscles. Left biceps biopsy is shown (Figures 15.2.1 and 15.2.2).

The most likely diagnosis is:

1. Inclusion body myositis
2. Polymyositis
3. Granulomatous myositis
4. Spinal muscular atrophy
5. CMT

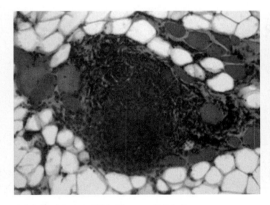

FIGURE 15.2.1 H & E stain (100x).

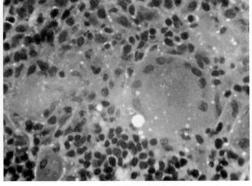

FIGURE 15.2.2 H & E stain (1000x).

DIAGNOSIS

- Muscle biopsy revealed multiple non-caseating granulomata that contained many multinucleated giant cells.
- Patients with chronic distal hand weakness are usually given different diagnoses such as carpal tunnel syndrome (CTS), cervical radiculopathy, arthritis, and so on, and it may take years before they see a neuromuscular specialist.
- The lack of sensory symptoms and the diffuse nature of the weakness suggested:
  - Myopathy
  - Motor neuron disease
  - Hirayama disease
  - Myasthenia gravis
- Creatine kinase (CK) elevation and myopathic EMG confirmed the diagnosis of distal myopathy and raised the following possibilities:
  - Hereditary myopathies
  - Inclusion body myositis
  - Myofibrillar myopathy
- Muscle biopsy reveals unexpected diagnosis. There was several non-caseating granulomas and endomyseal inflammation.
- Granulomatous myopathy is a rare form of inflammatory muscle disease:
  - It may present as progressive proximal weakness along with myasthenia gravis (MG) and thymoma.
  - Or it may present as a chronic distal weakness as a manifestation of sarcoidosis.
  - Frequently, search for sarcoidosis is not productive and the diagnosis of idiopathic granulomatous myopathy is given.
  - Prognosis is not good and, unfortunately, response to immunosupression or modulation is poor in the distal form.
  - Unlike the proximal variant, the distal idiopathic type does not affect the heart but it may extend to the proximal muscles.

REFERENCE

Jasim S, Shaibani A. Nonsarcoid granulomatous myopathy: two cases and a review of literature. *Int J Neurosci.* 2013 Jul;123(7):516–520.

CASE 15.3: A POLICEMAN WHO COULD NOT PULL THE TRIGGER

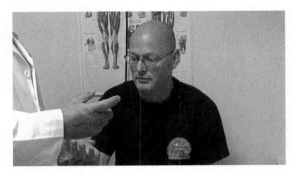

VIDEO 15.3

A 50-year-old police officer noticed 3 years earlier difficulty pulling the trigger. Gradually he developed difficulty dancing and swallowing. His mother was diagnosed with facioscapulo-humeral muscular dystrophy (FSHD) due to facial and leg weakness. Two aunts and two cousins were diagnosed with limb girdle muscular dystrophy (LGMD). One of them had congestive heart failure. CPK level was 124 U/L, and EMG revealed mixed short and long duration potentials in distal and proximal muscles of all extremities. Left biceps biopsy revealed chronic myopathic changes with no inflammation. Desmin staining was normal. Rare red-rimmed vacuoles were noted.

The following gene mutation analysis would be most appropriate:

1. GNE
2. Myosin
3. Desmin
4. PABPN1
5. FSHD

DIAGNOSIS

- The pattern of weakness (quadriceps, finger flexors, and feet extensors weakness), the chronicity and red-rimmed vacuoles (RRV) suggested inclusion body myositis. The age of the patient and the family history suggested hereditary inclusion body myositis (hIBM).
- Rimmed vacuoles are not specific and can be seen in:
  - IBM: sporadic and hereditary types
  - Oculopharyngeal muscular dystrophy (OPMD)
  - Oculopharyngodistal muscular dystrophy
  - Welander myopathty
  - Finnish-Markesbery myopathy
  - Distal muscular dystrophies
  - Distal myopathy with vocal cord weakness (MPD2)
- IBM subtypes:
  - Sporadic: IBM
  - IBM1 (myofibrillar myopathy)
  - IBM2 (GNG mutation)
  - IBM3: Joint contractures and ophthalmoplegia
  - IBM + paget dementia
- Hereditary IBM type 1:
  - Desminopathy, chromosome 2q35, dominant
  - Onset: 25–40 years
  - Quadriceps weakness and foot dorsiflexion weakness
  - Slow progression
  - Normal or mildly elevated CK
  - RRV and myopathic changes
- IBM2 (GNE) mutation is autosomal recessive and causes high CK and it usually spares quadriceps.
- Even sporadic IBM has a genetic component. Polymorphism in the TOMM40 gene modifies the risk of sIBM and the age of onset.

REFERENCES

Dalakas MD, et al. Desmin myopathy, a skeletal myopathy with cardiomyopathy caused by mutations in the desmin gene. *NEJM*. 2000 Mar 16;342(11):770–780.

Mastaglia FL, et al. Polymorphism in the TOMM40 gene modifies the risk of developing sporadic inclusion body myositis and the age of onset of symptoms. *Neuromuscul Disord*. 2013 Dec;23(12):969–974.

CASE 15.4: "FISH MOUTH" HANDSHAKE AND FACIAL WEAKNESS

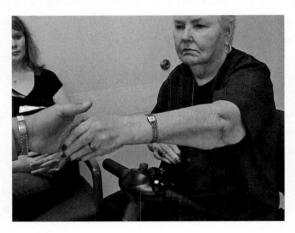

VIDEO 15.4

A 67-year-old woman presented with a 5-year history of gait imbalance and dysphagia. Examination is shown. CPK was 800 U/L, and EMG revealed mixed short and long duration potentials in the proximal and distal arm and leg muscles bilaterally. Discontinuation of atorvastatin and treatment with oral steroids reduced the CK to 300 and led to improvement of the stamina for a couple of months. No objective changes in the muscle strength were noted.

Regarding the case:

1. CK reduction with steroids argues against IBM.
2. The disease is due to statins.
3. Statins may have worsened weakness produced by IBM.
4. She is a good candidate for intravenous immunoglobulin (IVIG).
5. The pattern of weakness is not typical for IBM.

DIAGNOSIS

- The practice of adjusting the dose of prednisone based on the CK level is not recommended, as steroids stabilize the cell membrane and reduce the CK level regardless of the cause.
  - Strength measurement is the most valid outcome measure in monitoring recovery of myopathies. The 6-min walk test has been the standard for assessing function in clinical trials.
- Statins can cause different kinds of myopathies, including necrotizing myopathy and autoimmune inflammatory myopathy, with positive antibodies against 3-hydroxy-3-methyl-glutaryl-CoA (HMG-Co A) reductase.
- Also statins may unmask an underlying metabolic or mitochondrial myopathy, as 30% of statin-induced myopathies showed evidence of an underlying metabolic defect such as carnitine palmitoyltransferase II (CPT II), myoadenylate deaminase (MAD), and phosphorylase deficiencies.
- Some of these myopathies may improve after discontinuation of the statins, but it may take several months for maximum recovery. Others need to be treated with steroids and or other immunosuppressive agents.
- An IBM phenotype is not reported in association with statins therapy. Myopathies may be worsened by statins, which are therefore not recommended in patients with muscle disease.
- The pattern of weakness in this case was very typical for IBM, which should be highly suspected just after shaking hand with the patient ("fish mouth" handshake appearance due to weakness of finger flexors).
- Neither IVIG nor prednisone, azathioprine, or many other immunomodulatory agents have proven to be effective in treating IBM.
  - Some authorities advocate 3 months of steroids therapy to patients who show a CK level of more than 20K and intense endomysial inflammation. In our experience, improvement, if it happens, is transient and steroids do not change the natural history of the disease.

CASE 15.5: A FISHERMAN WHO COULD NOT PEEL SHRIMP ANY MORE

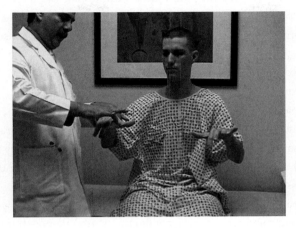

VIDEO 15.5

A 21-year-old shrimp peeler had developed weakness of his fingers 5 years earlier, which progressed to a degree that was not compatible with his job. He had no neck pain, arm numbness, dysphagia, or muscle twitching. Family history was non-relevant. Examination is shown. CPK was 530 U/L, and EMG revealed chronic diffuse denervation of the arm muscles with normal sensory and motor responses. EMG of the legs was normal.

The most likely diagnosis is:

1. Amyotrophic lateral sclerosis (ALS)
2. Hirayama disease (HD)
3. Inclusion body myositis (IBM)
4. West Nile virus infection
5. Cervical radiculopathy

DIAGNOSIS

- Chronic unilateral or bilateral pure motor weakness of the hand muscles in a young patient is not common. Differential diagnosis:
  - Cervical cord pathology such as syringomyelia: dissociated sensory loss is typically present
  - Brachial plexus pathology: sensory findings are usually present
  - Motor neurons disease: ALS, spinal muscular atrophy (SMA)
  - Distal myopathies
- Cervical spines are usually investigated before neuromuscular referrals are made.
- The lack of pain, radicular or sensory symptoms, and normal sensory nerve action potentials (SNAPS) and cervical magnetic resonance imaging (MRIs) ruled out most of the mentioned possibilities except:
  - Distal myopathy (usually not unilateral) and spinal muscular atrophy.
- EMG/NCS (electromyogram/nerve conduction study) demonstration of chronic distal denervation with normal sensory responses and no demyelinating features limited the diagnosis to motor neuron disease (MND).
- Segmental denervation pattern further narrowed the diagnosis to Hirayama disease (HD).
- HD is a sporadic and focal form of SMA that affects predominantly males at age 15–25 years.
  - Weakness and atrophy usually start unilaterally in C8-T1 muscles of the hand and forearm, typically in the dominant hand.
  - In a third of cases, the other hand is affected, and weakness may spread to the proximal muscles.
  - Deep tenson reflexes (DTRs) are normal or brisk, unlike most SMA cases where the reflexes are decreased or absent.
  - After progressive course of 6 years or less, the progression plateaus.
  - Extreme exacerbation of weakness in the cold and focal hyperhidrosis are reported.
  - The disease is more common in India.
  - Hypothesis: radiological forward displacement of the cervical dural sac and compressive flattening of the cervical cord during flexion suggest that this is a form of cervical myelopathy. The resulting ischemia leads to preferential damage of the motor neurons. Decompressive surgery is unlikely to be effective due to the chronic nature of the neurological insult.

REFERENCE

Hirayama K, Tokumaru Y. Cervical dural sac and spinal cord in juvenile muscular atrophy of distal upper extremity. *Neurology*. 2000;54:1922–1926.

CASE 15.6: A WRIST DROP AFTER A LONG FLIGHT

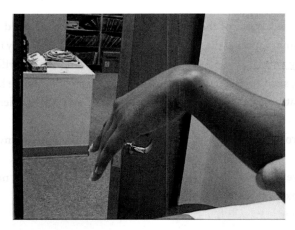

VIDEO 15.6

A 25-year-old woman presented with painless left wrist drop, which occurred after a 22-hour flight. She was stressed due to the fact that she had never lived away from her family, and she was crying during the examination.

The preservation of extension at the distal interphalangeal joins:

1. Suggests a psychogenic etiology
2. Is typically seen in radial neuropathy
3. Suggests brachial plexopathy
4. Rules out C7 radiculopathy
5. Suggests distal myopathy (Welander type)

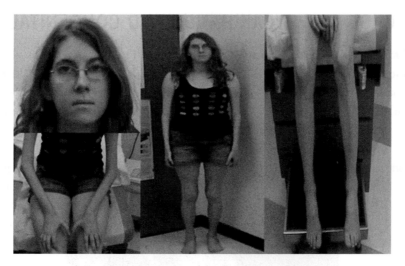

FIGURE 15.7.1 Patients photos showing wasting of the distal arm and leg muscles.

DIAGNOSIS

Severe hand weakness with cataract and ovarian agenesis:

Neuromuscular clinics sometimes receive enigmatic cases that defy diagnosis by the available tests. These cases are opportunities for the neuromuscular specialist to think creatively, looking for explanations.

- Involvement of multiple systems is seen in amyloidosis, vasculitis, and mitochondrial disorders.
- Cataract, ovarian agenesis, and seizures suggested a chromosomal disorder but chromosomal microarray was normal.
- In this case, the EMG suggested a chronic myopathic process, although motor neuron disorder could not be excluded. Muscle biopsy was not helpful due to the end stage nature of the disease process.
- Urine organic acid analysis revealed high level of 3-methylglutaconic acid with normal 3 hydroxyisovaleric acid.
- Mitochondrial genetic studies detected abnormal POLG. POLG sequencing revealed a heterozygous variant, c.2851T>A (p.Y951N), which was predicted to be deleterious.
- POLG mutations are heterogenous genetically and clinically. Neuromuscular manifestations of POLG mutations include:
  - Progressive external ophthalmoplegia
  - Neuropathy, ataxia, and retinitis pigmentosa (NARP)
  - Myoclonic epilepsy, myopathy sensory ataxia (MEMSA)
  - Mitochondrial spinocerebellar ataxia and epilepsy (MSCAE)

REFERENCE

Bekheirina MR, et al. POLG mutation in a patient with cataracts, early-onset distal muscle weakness and atrophy, ovarian dysgenesis and 3-methylglutaconic aciduria. *Gene*. 2012;499(1):209–212.

CASE 15.8: FINGER FLEXOR WEAKNESS AND QUADRICEPS SPARING

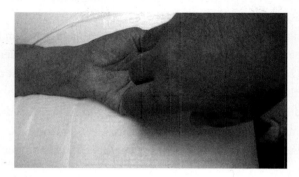

VIDEO 15.8

A 71-year-old woman presented with a 4-year history of gradually increasing inability to twist jar lids and difficulty swallowing water. Her quadriceps and facial muscles were normal. CK level was 283 U/L. EMG revealed evidence of irritative myopathy. Left biceps biopsy is shown (Figures 15.8.A and 15.8.B).

According to the IBM diagnostic criteria, this case qualifies for the diagnosis of:

1. Definite IBM
2. Probable IBM
3. Possible IBM
4. No IBM
5. None of the above

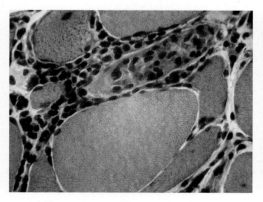

FIGURE 15.8A (400x).

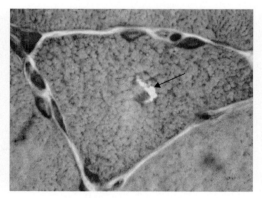

FIGURE 15.8B (100x).

DIAGNOSIS

- Muscle biopsy showed evidence of inflammatory myopathy (A) with red-rimmed vacuoles (RRVs) (B).
- There are at least 12 sets of diagnostic criteria for IBM; none of them is validated for sensitivity and specificity. At best, the most liberal of these criteria identifies 75% of cases clinically and 25% pathologically at the time of diagnosis. The most commonly used are the Griggs criteria.
- The presented case did not fulfill all the pathological criteria. It did show invasion of non-necrotic fibers with mononuclear cells and RRVs, but Congo red staining and EM examination were not done to look for congophilic material and nuclear or cytoplasmic inclusions.
  - ◆ The clinical criteria were met, including disease duration, the presence of proximal and distal weakness, and slightly elevated CK.
  - ◆ Quadriceps weakness is not required as long as there is finger flexor weakness or wrist flexor weakness.
  - ◆ There is no category for "probable IBM" in Griggs criteria (see supplement on page 617).
  - ◆ This is a case of possible IBM.

REFERENCE

Griggs RC, et al. Inclusion body myositis and myopathies. *Ann Neurol.* 1995;38:705.

CASE 15.9: DYSPHAGIA AND HAND GRIP WEAKNESS

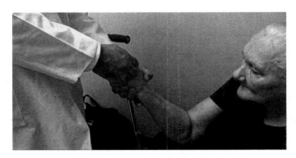

VIDEO 15.9

A 70-year-old woman presented with a 5-year history of right hand grip weakness that spread to the left hand after 2 years. She then developed dysphagia and weight loss. The leg muscle strength was normal. CK level was 450 U/L. EMG showed many short and long duration units in the biceps and wrist flexors.

The combination of chronic facial weakness, dysphagia, and distal arm weakness is typically seen in:

1. Inclusion body myositis (IBM)
2. Facioscapulohumeral muscular dystrophy (FSHD)
3. Myotonic dystrophy (DM)
4. Polymyositis (PM)
5. Amyotrophic lateral sclerosis (ALS)

DIAGNOSIS

- Despite the hectic schedule of the neuromuscular clinics, there is time for fun. Some patients have a good sense of humor and turn frustration into hope, while others find the time to celebrate their improvement by showing some funny talents.
- This Vietnam veteran had traumatic paraplegia and had been wheelchair bound for years. He developed compression of bilateral ulnar nerves at the elbows from excessive use of the arms to propel himself. He tried to show appreciation of our service by showing us a talent that he and his dog "Damn Good" mastered over the years and that had become their main source of income.
- Ulnar nerve is vulnerable to compression at the elbow because it travels through a narrow space (cubital tunnel) with little support. C8 radiculopathy also causes pain along the ulnar side of the arm and atrophy of FDI. Atrophy of thenar muscles and denervation of non ulnar C8 muscles are not features of ulnar neuropathy.
- Arthritis and repetitive elbow flexion are the main risk factors, but in the majority of cases, no clear cause is found for compression. It is more common in diabetics with neuropathy due to increased vulnerability of nerves to pressure. PTS typically affect upper trunk.
- Avoidance of pressure on the elbow and elbow support are to be tried first.
- Surgery is indicated if there is wasting of the intrinsic hand muscles or if the compression is severe.
- Cubital tunnel release and medial nerve transposition are the main surgical techniques. They are equally effective.

REFERENCE

Calliandro P, et al. Treatment of ulnar neuropathy at the elbow. *Cochrane Database Sys Rev.* 2011 Feb;16(2).

CHAPTER 16

DISTAL LEG WEAKNESS

CASE 16.1: FEET PAIN AND POSTURAL SYNCOPE

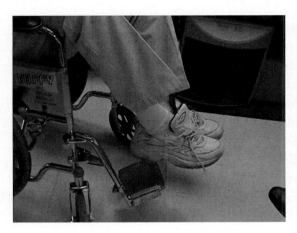

VIDEO 16.1

A 66-year-old man presented with a 3-year history of severe burning sensation in the feet and loss of balance. He then developed hand numbness and postural lightheadedness. He fainted once when he stood up fast. A year later he lost weight due to diarrhea. His examination revealed moderate proximal and distal weakness, right foot drop, distal sensory impairment, and diffuse areflexia. He older brother and father had similar symptoms. Electromyogram (EMG) revealed mixed axonal and demyelinating neuropathy. Also he had moderate bilateral focal median nerve lesion at the wrists. Cerebrospinal fluid (CSF) protein was normal. Due to the progression of the illness and the lack of explanation, he had a left sural nerve biopsy.

Which of the following stains/preparations would be most useful for the diagnosis?

1. Modified trichrome
2. Congo red stain viewed under polarized light
3. Hematoxylin and eosin (H & E) stain
4. Semithin sections
5. Teased nerve fiber preparation

What diagnosis is suggested by the combination of the following findings:

1. Family history
2. Dysautonomia features
3. Bilateral carpal tunnel syndrome (CTS)
4. Painful neuropathy
5. Progressive course

DIAGNOSIS

Familial amyloid polyneuropathy (FAP):

- Nerve biopsy revealed green birefringent deposits when Congo red-stained tissue was visualized under polarized light. Mutation analysis revealed Transthyretin mutation diagnostic of a form of familial amyloid neuropathy (FAP).
- Amyloid is a misfolded insoluble protein that cannot be digested and degraded and therefore it accumulates in the tissue and damages them. It can be systemic or localized to certain organs.
- The most vulnerable tissues are nerves, autonomic ganglia, kidney, gastrointestinal (GI) tract, and heart.
  - Familial amyloidosis is usually autosomal dominant and is caused by mutation of TTR, apolipoprotein A1, or gelsoline.
  - Primary amyloidosis (AL amyloidosis) is caused by deposition of immunoglobin G (IG) light chains. It could be part of lymphoma, multiple myeloma, other lymphoproliferative disorders or without a clear cause.
- The triad of dysautonomia (usually presents as postural hypotension), severe CTS (hand numbness), and painful feet (polyneuropathy) is highly suspicious of FAP, especially if there is a family history or nerve conduction study (NCS) evidence of axonal polyneuropathy.
- Diagnosis is made by the finding of apple green birefringent deposits in the nerve tissue, abdominal fat, or rectal biopsy. These deposits do not react to antibodies to light chains (unlike AL amyloidosis) but to antibodies to TTR, gelsoline, or apolipoprotein A1.
- TTR mutation is the most common FAP, and it occurs in two phenotypes:
  - FAP I: develops in the third to fourth decades. CTS is not severe but feet pain and hypotension are severe. Renal and cardiac involvement is common.
  - FAP II: Milder form with more severe CTS and less severe dysautonomia and renal/cardiac involvement. It appears in the seventies and the patients have long survival.
- Abdominal fat aspiration, if done from at least two sites, is probably as sensitive as nerve biopsy to detect amyloid deposits.
- Blood test for mutations of TTR, apolipoprotine A1, and gelsoline is advised to characterize this familial disorder further.

CASE 16.2: ASYMMETRIC PAINFUL FOOT DROP

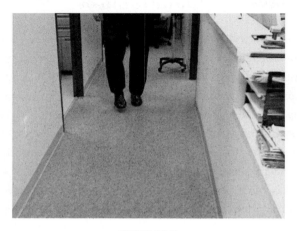

VIDEO 16.2

A 54-year-old man with a 3-month history of severe feet pain that started in the left side. He then developed hand numbness and proximal leg weakness and weight loss. Sed rate was 25 mm/hour and antinuclear antibodies (ANA) were negative. EMG revealed axonal polyneuropathy. CSF protein was 75mg/dl. Nerve biopsy pictures are shown (Figures 16.2.1, 16.2.2).

The pathological picture confirms the diagnosis of:

1. Amyloidosis
2. Vasculitis of the peripheral nervous system (PNS)
3. Sarcoidosis
4. Chronic inflammatory demyelinating polyneuropathy (CIDP)
5. Leprosy

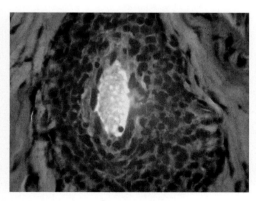

FIGURE 16.2.1 H&E stain: 400x.

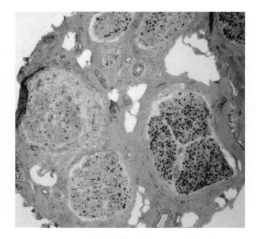

FIGURE 16.2.2 Modified Gromori Trichorme stain: 100x.

DIAGNOSIS

- Foot drop is commonly seen in neuromuscular clinics. It can be caused by polyneuropathy, peroneal neuropathy, L5 radiculopathy, lumbosacral plexopathy, and certain myopathies and myasthenia gravis (MG).
- Painful neuropathy is commonly seen in amyloidosis, vasculitis, familial autonomic and sensory neuropathy, and diabetes mellitus.
- Progressive asymmetrical painful neuropathy with asymmetrical foot drop should always raise the possibility of vasculitis, which could be systemic in the context of viral infections, connective tissue disease, malignancy, and so on, or isolated to the PNS (non-systemic vasculitis). In these cases, a nerve biopsy is indicated, as it would be the only way to confirm the diagnosis.
- Nerve biopsy findings diagnostic of vasculitis are reported in 50% of cases, but partial findings can be useful in the right clinical context.
- There are no clinical trials on treatment of isolated PNS vasculitis, but the standard therapy is a combination of steroids and intravenous (IV) or oral cyclophosphamide. The response rate is high, but 30% of cases relapse and some cases develop chronic feet pain even after resolution of vasculitis.
- Nerve biopsy findings of vasculitis:
  - Endoneurial and perineurial inflammation and mural infiltration with mononuclear inflammatory cells (Figure 16.2)
  - Eosinophils may predominate the inflammatory infiltrate in some cases of systemic vasculitis (i.e., Churg-Strauss syndrome and Wagner granulomatosis)
  - Fibrinoid necrosis of the small endoneurial blood vessels
  - Thrombosis, obliteration of lumen
  - Differential fascicular degeneration (Figure 16.2.2) and recanalization (chronic cases)
- Combined nerve and muscle and may be skin biopsy, increase the diagnostic yield. In patients with foot drop, superficial peroneal nerve and peroneus brevis muscle biopsy is appropriate. In other cases, sural nerve and gastrocnemius muscle biopsy is equally productive.

CASE 16.3: FAMILIAL DISTAL WEAKNESS

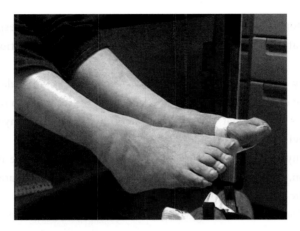

VIDEO 16.3

A 66-year-old woman presented with bilateral foot drop and wrists extensor weakness evolved over 5 years with no sensory symptoms or signs. Deep tendon reflexes (DTRs) were absent diffusely, and proximal strength was normal. There was no facial weakness. She had three children with similar symptoms. Sural responses were normal. EMG revealed chronic distal denervation of the lower and upper extremities and low motor amplitude.

The most likely diagnosis is:

1. Charcot-Marie-Tooth (CMT) disease
2. Spinal muscular atrophy (SMA)
3. Lead poisoning
4. Diphtheria
5. Vasculitis

DIAGNOSIS

- As in other branches of medicine, careful observation and sound reasoning are crucial for the right diagnosis and to save patients unnecessary procedures.
- Sequential foot drop in this patient suggested vasculitis, but the lack of feet pain and the preservation of the sural responses and ankle reflexes and the focal conduction block of the peroneal nerves at the fibular heads suggested compressive lesions at the knees.
- The patient was not aware of the importance of the recliner in causing her symptoms and therefore she did not volunteer to mention it. Only when she was questioned did she gave the mentioned history. She was advised to quit using the recliner, and her peroneal neuropathy recovered completely within 6 weeks.
- Compression of the peroneal nerves is common in patients with polyneuropathy, especially diabetic neuropathy and alcoholic neuropathy, but in this case there is no evidence of polyneuropathy.
- L5 Radiculopathy is ruled out by having normal tibialis posterior EMG and non-remarkable LS MRI.
- If conduction block was seen in other sites, especially in non at risk patients, one had to look for HNPP.

CASE 16.5: RIGHT FOOT DROP AND INFLAMMATORY MUSCLE BIOPSY

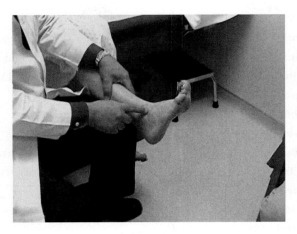

VIDEO 16.5

A 61-year-old woman presented with the shown findings. Creatine kinase (CK) level was 650 U/L. The most appropriate next testing is:

1. Muscle biopsy
2. Facioscapulohumeral muscular dystrophy (FSHD) mutation analysis
3. Lumbar spine magnetic resonance imaging (LS MRI)
4. Emerin gene mutation analysis
5. Nerve conduction study (NCS)

What diagnosis is suggested by the combination of the following findings:

1. Asymmetric onset
2. Distal weakness
3. Scapular winging
4. Facial weakness
5. Inflammatory pathology

DIAGNOSIS

Myopathic foot drop:

- Painless asymmetrical foot drop, scapular winging, and myopathic EMG suggest facioscapulohumeral muscular dystrophy (FSHD). Neurogenic and myopathic scapulo-peroneal syndrome is also possible. This patient had contraction of D4Z4 allele, confirming the diagnosis of FSHD.
- Unilateral or bilateral foot drop may be caused by muscle disease.
- Factors that would suggest a myopathic etiology include:
  - Preserved bulk or even compensatory hypertrophy of the extensor digitorum brevis (EDB) due to the lack of involvement of the intrinsic foot muscles, unlike neurogenic etiology when these muscles are affected early
  - The lack of sensory symptoms or signs
  - The lack of feet pain
  - Preservation of sural responses
  - Lack of denervation of the tibialis anterior; spontaneous activity may be seen as a part of irritative myopathy
  - The presence of other features of muscle disease like proximal weakness and scapular winging
- FSHD is a common inherited muscle disease where tibialis anterior muscles are affected early, leading to unilateral or bilateral foot drop usually in association with scapular winging and facial weakness. Twenty percent of cases do not show facial weakness.
- Foot drop can be the presenting symptom of FSHD, which may lead to diagnostic confusion with peroneal neuropathy and L5 radiculopathy and sometimes amyotrophic lateral sclerosis (ALS).
- Affected family members may not be aware of their myopathic features, and their examination is usually helpful.
- Asymmetry can be striking, leading to unilateral foot drop or facial weakness.
- Inflammation in the muscle biopsy is characteristic, leading to misdiagnosis as polymyositis. Muscle biopsy is not required for the diagnosis, which can be made from a blood sample.
- 20% of patients end up in a wheelchair.

CASE 16.6: CALVES ATROPHY AND MODERATELY HIGH CK LEVEL

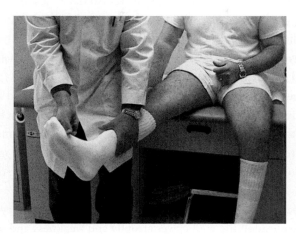

VIDEO 16.6

A 30-year-old man presented who had difficulty walking on his toes at age 15 years. At that time he was found to have a CK level of 2,800 U/L, and EMG revealed fibrillations in the bilateral calf muscles. He was diagnosed with axonal neuropathy. Gradually, he developed more atrophy of the calves, proximal leg and arm weakness, and weakness of the finger flexors. CK level was 3,000–4,000 U/L, and NCS were normal. EMG revealed irritative myopathy involving proximal and distal muscles of the arms and legs. There was no family history of muscle disease. He started using a walker 7 years after the onset of the symptoms. Left biceps biopsy revealed chronic inflammatory myopathic changes.

The most appropriate immunohistochemical testing on the muscle biopsy is:

1. CD4/CD8 antibodies
2. Dysferlin antibodies
3. Dystrophin antibodies
4. Sarcoglycan antibodies
5. Calpain antibodies

DIAGNOSIS

- Distal myopathy is a feature of many myopathic disorders; most of them are hereditary.
- Among the sporadic disorders, inclusion body myositis (IBM) is the most common myopathy with distal involvement.
- Dystrophic myopathies like myotonic dystrophy usually cause distal weakness, along with facial and proximal weakens.
- There is a group of hereditary myopathies that are characterized by distal weakness only, at least in the beginning of the disease. These disorders lack molecular understanding and they are classified according to the region affected, mode of inheritance, and age of onset. Many of them are allelic to specific limb girdle muscular dystrophy (LGMDs). More molecular understanding will likely change the classification in the future.
- Miyoshi myopathy is one of the better characterized distal hereditary myopathies.
  - It starts in early adult life with calves atrophy and weakness and remarkably elevated CK level and myopathic EMG.
  - It is caused by mutation of dysferlin gene and is allelic with LGMD 2B.
  - Endomysial inflammation in muscle biopsy may lead to erroneous diagnosis of polymyositis.
- Patients with myopathic calves atrophy do not need a muscle biopsy unless mutation analysis carried on white blood cells (WBC) fails to reveal absent dysferlin staining.

CASE 16.7: CALVES ATROPHY AND MILD CK ELEVATION

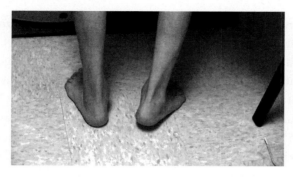

VIDEO 16.7

A 53-year-old man presented with resting painful cramping of the calf muscles since age 20 years. He noticed the inability to stand on his toes 25 years earlier. There was severe atrophy and weakness of the calf muscles. Hip flexors were slightly weak. Arm muscles were 5/5. Reflexes were brisk except for the ankles, which were absent; sensation and sural responses were normal, but the compound muscle action potentials (CMAPs) were low. Creatine kinase (CK) level was 420 U/L and EMG Showed large motor units potentials (MUPs) with an amplitude of 12-15mV and a firing frequency of 20-30 HZ in the arms and legs and thoracic paraspinal muscles (TPS) muscles.

The cause of the calves' weakness in this case is likely:

1. Myioshi myopathy
2. Spinal muscular atrophy (SMA)
3. Amyotrophic lateral sclerosis (ALS)
4. Bilateral S1 radiculopathy
5. LS plexopathy

DIAGNOSIS

- Chronic progressive distal weakness that starts in the legs is an important scenario in neuromuscular clinics.
- NCS/EMG play a crucial role to sort out neurogenic from myopathic conditions.
- Mild CK elevation frequently leads to confusion with myopathy, but it is a common finding in denervating conditions like motor neuron disorders.
- In the elderly, it is important to rule out spinal pathology such as severe spondylosis resulting in LS polyradiculopathy, although the lack of pain is atypical.
- Muscle biopsy is not necessary in neurogenic cases; if done, it would show chronic denervation and re-innervation.
- In spinal muscular atrophy, loss of DTRs in the affected limbs is expected. Hyperreflexia occurs in 10% of cases. Pes Cavus is common.
- Familial ALS and neuronal CMT are important considerations.
- Most SMAs manifests themselves during infancy and childhood, but some present in adulthood.
- Some distal SMAs in adults are reported in only one or two families, and their genetic pattern varies from AD to AR and even X-linked recessive modes. All of them are slowly progressive and usually they spare cranial nerves.
- Adult onset distal SMAs or hereditary motor neuropathies (HMNs):
  - HMN 2A: Autosomal dominant 12q24.3; some with vocal fold and diaphragm weakness
  - HMN 2B Autosomal dominant/recessive.7q11.23
  - Distal SMA, X-linked Xq12–q13
  - Distal SMA 3 (DSMA 3):Chromosome 11q13.3; recessive

REFERENCE

Wee CD, et al. The genetics of SMA. *Curr Opin Neurol.* 2010, October;23:450–458.

CASE 16.8: CHRONIC CALVES ATROPHY

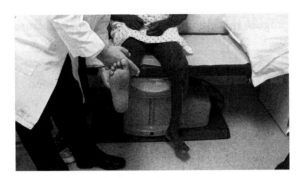

VIDEO 16.8

A 52-year-old man was an avid runner until 18 years earlier, when he had difficulty running, and gradually he developed atrophy of the distal leg muscles. Examination revealed weakness of plantar flexors and extensors with normal sensation and absent ankle reflexes. CPK level was 320 IU/L. LS MRI revealed mild degenerative charges. He had seven healthy siblings. EMG revealed diffuse chronic denervation with MUPs of 15 mV amplitude and 20 msec duration in all the tested muscles.

Mutation responsible for this disease is likely located on the following chromosome:

1. 7
2. 12
3. X
4. 22
5. 14

DIAGNOSIS

- The biopsy shows muscle tissues stained with nonspecific esterase that is used to delineate denervated fibers. There were many small dark angulated fibers (moderate denervation).
- Unilateral or bilateral calf hypertrophy or pseudohypertrophy may be caused by:
  - Muscle disease: dystrophinopathy, amyloid myopathy, sarcoid myopathy
  - Nerve hyperexcitability: neuromyotonia
  - Nerve root irritation: S1 radiculopathy
- In this case, since the last possibility is very rare and the CK elevation was more than expected for that cause, a muscle biopsy was necessary to rule out other causes.
- As a rule, radiculopathy causes muscle atrophy, but for poorly understood reasons, hypertrophy can occur. Continuous discharge of the affected nerve root due to irritation is a possible explanation.

REFERENCE

Swartz KR, Fee DB, Trost GR, Waclawik AJ. Unilateral calf hypertrophy seen in lumbosacral stenosis: case report and review of the literature. *Spine* (Phila Pa 1976). 2002 Sep 15;27(18):E406–E409.

CASE 17.6: CALVES ATROPHY

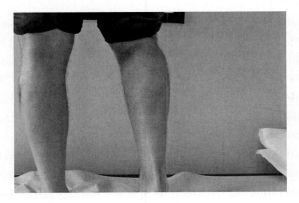

VIDEO 17.6

A 54-year-old man presented with a 15-year history of inability to stand on his toes. He had difficulty buttoning shirts. There was no significant family history. In addition to what is shown in the examination, the rest of the muscles were 5/5. There was calves atrophy. Sensation was intact and sural responses were normal. CK level was 390 U/L. EMG revealed mixed short and long duration motor unit potentials in the calf muscles with no spontaneous activity. Genetic testing for CMT and SMA were negative. Left gastrocnemius biopsy showed dystrophic non-inflammatory myopathy.

The following typically cause(s) calves atrophy:

1. Dysferlinopathy
2. Telithinopathy (LGMD2G)
3. Desminopathy
4. Calpainopathy
5. Dystrophinopathy

DIAGNOSIS

- Inability to walk on toes is characteristic of involvement of the posterior compartment muscles of the forelegs. When chronic, patients consider it as normal and not functionally disturbing, and thus do not seek medical advice. They are usually referred due to abnormal CK level.
- Absence of ankle reflexes, in addition to the distal weakness and the presence of family history, may lead to diagnostic confusion with hereditary motor neuropathy and distal spinal muscular atrophy.
- Mild CK elevation is not unusual in denervating conditions and therefore it may not raise a suspicion of myopathy. Mixed (short and long duration) motor unit potentials can occur in chronic denervation and in chronic myopathies and may add to the confusion.
- Muscle biopsy is useful in early stages by showing denervation changes (group atrophy in chronic cases) in neurogenic disease and chronic myopathic or dystrophic changes in myopathic disease.
- In severe cases, end stage pathology does not help this differentiation. Immunostaining on even a few remaining fibers may help to sort out cases of dysferlinopathy and desminopathy. Genetic testing for these disorders in the blood or muscle is helpful.
- In this case, CK level was too low for dysferlinopathy and desmin staining should be attempted.
- Myofibrillar myopathy (desminopathy) is a heterogeneous group of disorders that usually cause distal weakness and cardiomyopathy.
- Dysferlinopathy and desminopathy typically cause calf atrophy. Dystrophinopathy and LGMD 2G typically cause calf hypertrophy.

REFERENCE

Bushby, KM. Making sense of limb girdle muscular dystrophy. *Brain*. 1999;122(8):1403–1420.

CASE 17.7: BIG CALVES AND REMARKABLY ELEVATED CK LEVEL

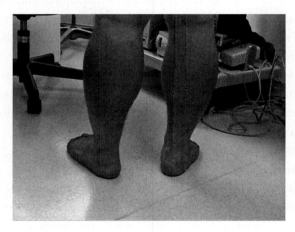

VIDEO 17.7

A 43-year-old man presented with difficulty standing on his toes, noticed 10 years earlier. He had mild quadriceps weakness and a CK level of 3,350. EMG showed mixed short and long duration potentials.

Calves hypertrophy is a feature of:

1. Becker muscular dystrophy (BMD)
2. Amyloid myopathy
3. Sarcoglycanopathy
4. Dysferlinopathy
5. Inclusion body myositis (IBM)

DIAGNOSIS

- Calves enlargement is an important feature of dystrophinopathies; it is due to fatty replacement rather than actual hypertrophy. It is also observed typically in amyloid myopathy and some sarcoglycanopathies, but not in IBM or dysferlinopathy, where calf atrophy is the rule.
- Dystrophin is a subsarcolemmal protein in the skeletal and cardiac muscles.
  - It stabilizes the membrane during muscle contraction and relaxation.
  - Abnormal level of dystrophin leads to loss of integrity of muscle fibers during contraction and relaxation, leading to membrane damage necrosis.
- Dystrophin gene is a large gene located on Xp21 but only less than 1% of gene codes for dystrophin (exons).
- Phenotype depends on the type of mutation (in frame or out of frame) and the quantity of functional dystrophin in the muscles rather than the site of mutation.
  - Less than 5% of the normal is associated with Duchenne muscular dystrophy (DMD).
  - 5%–20% of normal correlates with the intermediate phenotype (mild DMD or severe BMD).
  - 20%–50% of normal is associated with mild to moderate BMD.
- Dystrophin gene mutations:
  - Large deletions: two-thirds of cases
  - Point mutations leading to stop codons: 5%–10%
  - Duplications: 5%
- Out of frame mutations lead to complete disruption of translation and result in a total loss of dystrophin: DMD
- In frame mutations: translation of dysfunctional protein: BMD phenotype
- Phenotypes of dystrophinopathy:
  - Duchenne muscular dystrophy (DMD)
  - Becker muscular dystrophy (BMD)
  - Myalgia
  - Myoglobinuria
  - Cardiomyopathy
  - HyperCKemia

CASE 17.8: CHRONIC DISTAL ARM DENERVATION

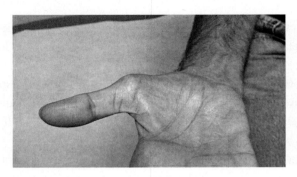

VIDEO 17.8

A 47-year-old man presented with a 13-year history of weakness and atrophy of the right hand muscles. Thoracic outlet syndrome surgery did not help. CK level and cerebrospinal fluid (CSF) examination were normal. Cervical MRI was normal Nerve conduction study (NCS) showed no conduction block. The compound muscle action potentials (CMAPs) of the right median and ulnar nerves were reduced. Sensory responses were normal. EMG revealed diffuse chronic denervation of the right arm muscles.

The lesion is likely located at the level of:

1. Motor neurons
2. Motor nerves
3. Brachial plexus
4. Axons
5. Myelin

DIAGNOSIS

- The presence of diffuse weakness and denervation that spans multiple nerve roots with preservation of sensory responses and reduced reflexes suggest a lower motor neuron lesion.
- Multifocal motor neuropathy with conduction block may present similarly, but the presence of conduction blocks and the lack of diffuse denervation would distinguish these cases. This patient was treated with intravenous immunoglobulin (IVIG), with no improvement, before being referred to our center.
- Cervical polyradiculopathy duo to an infiltrative lesion of the motor nerve root such as lymphoma is possible, but the long duration and normal cervical MRI ruled out this possibility.
- ALS may start with focal lower motor neuron signs but it usually spreads to other muscles and evolves into a typical picture within a year or two. Distal spinal muscular atrophy is usually bilateral and distal.
- Chronic focal lower motor neuron disease (Hirayama disease, monomelic amyotrophy) is well known.
  - It is sporadic and affects males 10 times more than females. Age of onset is 13–15 years.
  - Starts with distal single limb weakness; right is twice as likely affected than left.
  - Subclinical involvement of the other arm is common, and in 10% of cases, proximal weakness is evident.
  - 40% of times it spreads to the other side. It progresses over 5 years and then plateus for decades.
  - Most denervation is in C8-T1 muscles but proximal and even lower extremities muscles may be affected. Cervical MRI: cord atrophy is seen in 30%–50% of cases.
  - It is speculated that posterior epidural venous plexus engorgement during flexion contributes to the pathology, but that does not explain the presence of denervation in the legs.

CHAPTER 18

HYPERREFLEXIA

CASE 18.1: JAW CLONUS

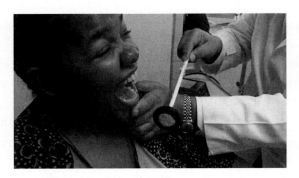

VIDEO 18.1

A 30-year-old woman developed dysarthria, progressive weakness, and hyperreflexia of the arms with normal sensation. Her brain magnetic resonance imaging (MRI) was normal. The tongue showed atrophy and fasciculations.

Which of the following disorders is typically associated with jaw clonus?

1. Amyotrophic lateral sclerosis (ALS)
2. Chronic inflammatory demyelinating polyneuropathy (CIDP)
3. Myotonic dystrophy
4. Progressive muscular atrophy
5. Spinal muscular atrophy

DIAGNOSIS

- Hyperreflexia is an important sign of upper motor neuron dysfunction.
- Hyperreflexia may be present in anxious persons.
- Even normoactive reflexes are considered to be abnormal when they are not expected to be there, for example, preserved knee reflexes in CIDP, preserved ankle reflexes in the face of severe feet numbness.
- The presence of Babinski and Hoffman signs support the pathological basis of hyperreflexia.
- The jaw jerk is often deleted from the neurological examination.
  - The jaw jerk is served by the trigeminal nerve for its afferent and efferent connections (unlike the blink and corneal reflexes, which are served by trigeminal and facial nerves).
  - A brisk jaw jerk indicates a lesion cephalad to mid pons, where the nerve emerges.
  - A combination of a brisk jaw jerk and tongue fasciculations is characteristic of ALS.
  - Grading of the jaw jerk follows the same medical research council (MRC) grading system that is used to grade other monosynaptic reflexes such as knee, biceps, triceps, and ankle reflexes.

CASE 18.2: SPASTIC DYSARTHRIA

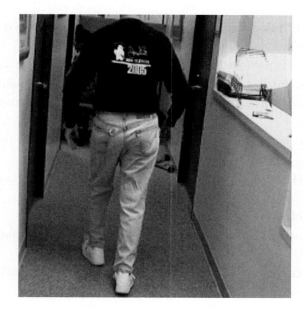

VIDEO 18.2

A 27-year-old man presented with dysarthria and spasticity of the arms and legs evolving over 5 years to complete disability. He had normal sensation and diffuse hyperreflexia. Tongue was weak but not atrophic. MRI of the brain and spinal cord and cerebrospinal fluid (CSF) examination were normal, and there was no denervation observed by electromyogram (EMG) study.

The most likely diagnosis is:

1. Multiple sclerosis
2. Primary lateral sclerosis
3. Hereditary spastic paraplegia
4. Tropical spastic paraplegia
5. Cerebrovascular disease

DIAGNOSIS

- This variant of ALS is the most difficult to diagnosis until later in the course and after other causes of myelopathy are ruled out.
- The most common presentation is progressive stiffness of the legs and poor balance.
- In some cases, slurring of speech can be subtle and may be confused with myasthenia gravis, especially when some patients report increasing fatigue toward the end of the day.
- Pseudobulbar palsy and hyperreflexia with increased tone in the extremities are common.
- Evolution to ALS occurs in more than 70% of cases with the appearance of fasciculations and atrophy.
- Other causes of non-compressive myelopathy are to be considered:
  1. Hereditary spastic paraplegia: the course is more chronic and family history may be present.
  2. Tropical spastic paraplegia: history of living in the tropics, abnormal CSF examination, and positive HTLV-1 antibodies.
  3. Adrenomyeloneuropathy: X-linked, abnormal MRI of the brain and spinal cord, increased very long chair fatty acids in the serum, and ABCD1 mutation is detected.
  4. B_{12} deficiency: presence of sensory symptoms, memory impairment, optic atrophy, macrocytic anemia, and low vitamin B_{12} level.
  5. Copper deficiency: sensory symptoms are common, but cases with purely motor symptoms with fasciculations have been reported. Leucopenia is common and serum copper level is low. Usually there is a history of gastrectomy years earlier.

CASE 18.3: INAPPROPRIATE CRYING AND LAUGHTER

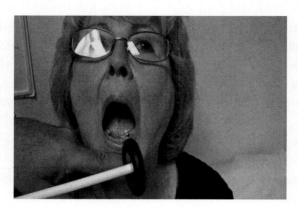

VIDEO 18.3

A 68-year-old woman presented with a 6-month history of inappropriate laughter and crying, cough, and slurring of speech.

Emotional lability or pseudobulbar affect (PBA) can occur in:

1. Amyotrophic lateral sclerosis (ALS)
2. Multiple sclerosis (MS)
3. Cerebral multi-infarct state
4. Traumatic brain injury (TBI)
5. Alzheimer disease

DIAGNOSIS

- Pathological laughter and crying (emotional incontinence) result from release of the physical components (reflexes) of these emotions from the inhibitory cortical control. Therefore, these patients experience outbursts of crying or laughter that are not triggered by appropriate stimuli. Emotions can be paradoxical, such as laughing at bad news.
- Corticobulbar tracts or their cortical neurons are the targets of pathological process leading to PBA.
- The most common causes of PBA are: ALS, MS, multi-infarct state, Alzheimer disease, brainstem tumors, and TBI.
- In this case, jaw hyperreflexia and the presence of tongue fasciculations suggested ALS.
- In ALS, PBA carries a poor prognosis since it is associated with bulbar dysfunction (dyspnea, dysphagia, sialorrhea, etc.).
- Patients with pure upper motor neuron lesion (primary lateral sclerosis) that starts in the suprabulbar pathways may impose a diagnostic dilemma until the evolution of more complete diagnostic picture.
- PBA can be socially devastating.
- Depression commonly occurs and complicates the clinical picture.
- PBA usually responds to tricyclic antidepressants.
  - Dextromethorphan/quinidine is approved by the FDA for this condition.
  - Transaminases and QT interval should be periodically checked while taking this medication.
- All the mentioned options can cause PBA.

REFERENCE

Shaibani AT, Sabbagh MN, Doody R. Laughter and crying in neurologic disorders. *Neuropsychiatry Neuropsychol Behav Neurol.* 1994;7:243–250.

CASE 18.4: PATELLAR CLONUS

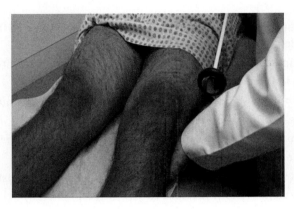

VIDEO 18.4

A 60-year-old man presented with poor balance and spastic gait starting 2 years earlier. He developed atrophy of the thigh muscles and twitching in the arms within a year. CK level was 350 U/L and the EMG study revealed widespread denervation of the tested legs and thoracic paraspinal muscles with normal sensory responses.

The cause of patellar clonus in this case is:

1. Myelopathy
2. Amyotrophic lateral sclerosis (ALS)
3. Multiple sclerosis (MS)
4. Spinal muscular atrophy
5. Myopathy

DIAGNOSIS

- Clonus is a series of involuntary rhythmic muscular contractions. It is usually initiated by tapping a tendon to generate a deep tendon reflex.
- The self-sustained contractions are due to the lack of central inhibition caused by upper motor neuron lesions, such as ALS, MS, stroke, and so on.
- Clonus corresponds to grade 4+ of deep tendon reflexes grading scale.
- Clonus is usually associated with spasticity.
- A fasciculation is a spontaneous discharge of a motor neuron cell or its axon and is a sign of lower motor neuron (LMN) lesion.
- The presence of myoclonus and fasciculations together is characteristic of ALS.
- Ankle and jaw clonus follows the same rules.
- Myoclonus is totally different from clonus. It is a sudden brief contraction of a muscle or a group of muscles. It is caused by a different group of central nervous system diseases such as encephalopathies or some forms of epilepsy.

CHAPTER 19

MUSCLE TWITCHING

CASE 19.1: PAINLESS MUSCLE TWITCHING

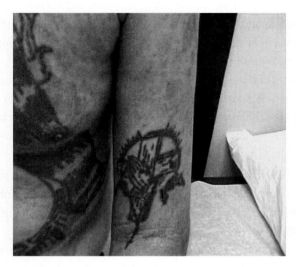

VIDEO 19.1

A 45-year-old man presented with a 1-year history of painless muscle twitching in the arms and chest, painful cramps in the arms, decreased muscle bulk, and weakness of the arms. DTRs were 3/4 and sensation was normal. Creatine kinase (CK) level was 345 U/L.

Comprehensive electromyogram (EMG) of this patient is expected to show:

1. Myokymia
2. Focal fasciculations
3. Neuromyotonia
4. Widespread fasciculations
5. Rippling muscle disease

DIAGNOSIS

- A fasciculation is a short-lived irregular spontaneous discharge of individual axons and:
  - Causes activation of all or part of muscle fibers that belong to a motor unit
  - Produces visible rippling of the involved muscle
- The old notion that fasciculations are generated only from motor neurons has been challenged. While motor neurons remain a possible origin (in ALS, for example), terminal axons seem to be the source in the majority of fasciculations (like benign fasciculation syndrome [BFS]).
- Fasciculations appear as single motor units in the needle EMG.
- Distal axonal fasciculations are more frequent than more proximal fasciculations (ALS) due to the short refractory period (3–4 msec) and short interspike intervals (5 msec).
- While spontaneous most of the time, fasciculations may be precipitated by percussion, activity, and cold.
- There is no relationship between fasciculations frequency and disease severity.
- Voluntary activity, unlike random fasciculations, is semi-rhythmic at a rate of 8 Hz.
  - Causes of fasciculations:
    - Peripheral nerve hyper-excitability disorder
    - Motor neuron diseases
    - Axonal neuropathies
    - Hyperthyroidism and hyperparathyroidism
    - Hypomagnesemia
    - Cholinergic overstimulation (OPC poisoning, pyridostigmine, etc.)
    - Hyperventilation (relative hypocalcaemia)
  - In amyotrophic lateral sclerosis (ALS), besides fasciculation, one may find fibrillations in many muscles, weakness, and hyperreflexia.
  - In BFS, there is no atrophy or weakness.
    - Serial examination is important to look for new onset weakness or atrophy or spread of the fasciculations in ALS
  - Fasciculations can be confused with tremor.

CASE 19.2: FACIAL TWITCHING

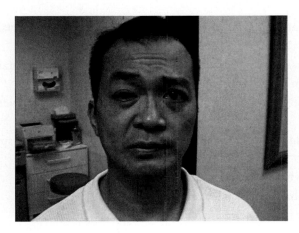

VIDEO 19.2

A 39-year-old man presented with involuntary recurrent blinking of the right eye. There was no facial weakness or numbness. Brain magnetic resonance imaging (MRI) was normal.

The most likely cause of this condition is:

1. Brainstem tumor
2. Aberrant vertebral artery
3. Stroke
4. Neuropathy
5. Amyotrophic lateral sclerosis (ALS)

DIAGNOSIS

- Involuntary intermittent twitching of muscles supplied by the facial nerve (hemifacial spasm).
- Hemifacial spasm is caused by compression of the facial nerve by a branch of the vertebro-basillar system at the base of the brain or by a tumor.
- Trauma to the nerve may produce the same (surgery on the facial nerve or previous Bell palsy).
- Periorbital and perioral muscles are affected, and sometimes the spasms spread to the other side.
- 5% of patients have a history of trigeminal neuralgia.
- Periodic botulinum toxin injections are very effective.
- For refractory cases, microvascular decompression is an option.

CASE 19.3: RHYTHMIC MUSCLE TWITCHING

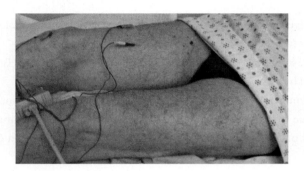

VIDEO 19.3

A 73-year-old man presented with generalized weakness and fatigue of 6 months duration. His examination revealed resting tremor of the hands, mild shuffling gait, and mild generalized weakness. The patient was referred to the neuromuscular clinic to be evaluated for "fasciculations of the thighs."

The recorded abnormal twitching of the right thing muscles is:

1. Fasciculations
2. Neuromyotonia
3. Voluntary movement
4. Tremor
5. Myoclonus

DIAGNOSIS

- In a progressively weak patient, especially if there is hyperreflexia, neurologists look for fasciculations to support the diagnosis of suspected ALS.
- Tremor in these cases is commonly confused with fasciculations. Hyperreflexia is commonly caused by anxiety and nervousness.
- Tongue and limbs tremor is common in the normal population. Action tremor is not hard to sort out due to its amelioration at rest. Resting tremor can be more confusing, especially when it occurs in proximal muscles and is not associated with other parkinsonian features.
- Weakness and atrophy along with fasciculation would support the diagnosis of ALS.
- Tremor is rhythmic while fasciculations are random. However, when fasciculations are frequent, tremor can be mimicked.
- Needle examination often helps to determine the rhythmicity of the discharges and their nature.

CASE 19.4: STRETCHING-INDUCED MUSCLE CONTRACTIONS

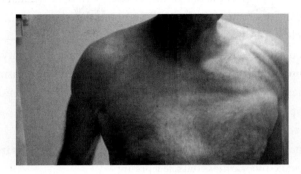

VIDEO 19.4

(courtesy of Michael Weiss, MD)

The patient is a 64-year-old man with a 3-year history of involuntary muscle movement, stiffness, and soreness. His clinical examination demonstrated normal muscle bulk and power. EMG was notable for electrical silence during the induced muscle contractions.

The demonstrated activity is:

1. Fasciculations
2. Myokymia
3. Rippling muscle
4. Tremor
5. Voluntary units

DIAGNOSIS

- The video shows rippling of the pectoralis muscles with stretching of the upper chest and shoulders, and percussion-induced muscle contractions.
- Rippling muscle syndrome is a rare disorder with multiple causes.
- The rippling muscles are electrically silent, suggesting that the activity is not generated by the muscle fibers but is due to calcium dysregulation by the endoplasmic reticulum.
- Touching or percussing the muscle usually triggers rippling.
- Hereditary rippling muscle syndrome:
  - Due to Caveolin mutations (LGMD 1C)
  - An autosomal dominant or recessive muscle disease that presents in the first 2 decades of life with wave-like painless muscle rippling
  - Proximal and or distal weakness and scapular winging
  - Muscle hypertrophy may happen
  - CK level is more than 10X normal
  - Muscle pathology: nonspecific myopathy with decreased Caveolin staining
- Sporadic rippling muscle syndrome:
  - Associated with myasthenia gravis (MG) or thymoma and it may precede their symptoms
  - Myalgia and mild CK elevation are common
  - Worsened by pyridostigmine
  - It may respond to immunosuppression

CASE 19.5: MUSCLE TWITCHING AND HYPERREFLEXIA

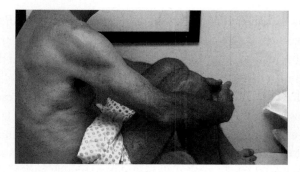

VIDEO 19.5

A 63-year-old man presented with a 6-month history of muscle twitching in the arms and mild weakness in the hand grips. His examination is shown. The EMG in the areas of profuse fasciculations showed only rare fasciculations and neurogenic motor unit potentials (MUPs) with firing frequency of 25 Hz diffusely. Fibrillations were rare.

On the prognosis of this disease:

1. 20% of patients live 5 years or more
2. 50% of patients live at least 3 years
3. 10% of patients survive more than 10 years
4. 10% of patients live less than 3 years
5. Bulbar involvement does not change the prognosis

DIAGNOSIS

- The video shows fasciculations in the arms clinically and by EMG and hyperreflexia.
- There are several sets of diagnostic criteria for ALS; all of them suffer from deficiency and miss at least 50% of cases in the time of diagnosis due to the fact that they are created as a research tool and not for clinical use.
- El Escorial criteria are the most commonly used and require the presence of evidence of progressive lower motor neuron (LMN) and upper motor neuron (UMN) degeneration in at least three regions (cranial, cervical, thoracic, and lumbar) for the definite diagnosis.
- Sometimes EMG evidence of active denervation lags behind and is replaced by chronic denervation potentials (high amplitude long duration units with high firing frequency) due to re-innervation. Almost always, with disease progression, active denervation appears and becomes widespread.
- Interestingly, needle examination of fasciculation-rich muscles usually shows much less electrical fasciculations than what is noticed clinically, even if the needle is inserted in the fasciculating area itself. The generators of fasciculations may be too deep for the needle to detect.
- Fasciculations are produced by "dying motor neurons" and, therefore, they are more frequent in the early stages of the disease; as the disease progresses, they are replaced by fibrillations and positive sharp waves (produced by motor neurons' death). One has to wait for at least 60 seconds with every needled examination before declaring the areas clean of fasciculation.
- Fifty percent of patients with Lou Gehrig disease (ALS) live at least three years after diagnosis; twenty percent live five years or more; and up to ten percent will survive more than ten years.
- Bulbar involvement is a bad prognostic sign.

CHAPTER 20

MUSCLE STIFFNESS AND CRAMPS

CASE 20.1A: SEVERE INTERMITTENT MUSCLE SPASMS

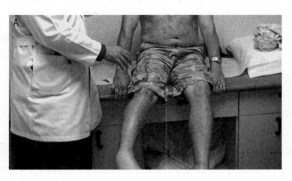

VIDEO 20.1A

A 39-year-old man with progressive stiffness of the back muscles starting a few months earlier, followed by severe intermittent sustained painful spasms of the legs and arms, which was triggered by painful stimuli, tapping the patella, or hearing a high-pitch sound. Creatine kinase (CK) level was 300U/L and electromyogram (EMG) revealed normal but continuous involuntary motor unit potentials. Voltage-gated potassium channel (VGKC) antibody titer was normal. Baclofen pump reduced the cramps by 80%.

Such severe painful muscle cramps that are triggered by stretching, emotions, and painful stimulation are seen in:

1. Stiff person syndrome (SPS)
2. Tetany
3. Tetanus
4. Myokymia
5. Myotonia

DIAGNOSIS

- Unlike peripheral causes of stiffness and spasms, central causes like SPS and tetanus are provoked by emotions and painful stimuli.
- Stiff person syndrome (SPS) usually presents with progressive stiffness and gait difficulty. In severe cases, severe painful cramps may be triggered by sensory stimulation and may produce fallings. They are usually bilateral and cause arms, legs, and trunk extension and feet inversion.
- Both agonist and antagonist muscles contract simultaneously. These contractions can be severe enough to cause fractures and disability. Startle response is usually augmented, but trismus is rare. SPS may be associated with seizures, thymoma, and myasthenia gravis. Anti Glutamic acid decarboxylase (GAD) antibodies are very high in 60%–90% of cases.
- Tetanus is caused by a toxin that is produced by clostridium tetani called tetanospasmin, which inhibits the release of glycine or gamma aminobutyric acid (GABA).
  - Full immunization against tetanus is 100% protective, but only 10% of Americans complete the series.
  - Acute wound infection is the major source.
  - Severe painful spasms can be localized or generalized, and the closer the wound to the head, the worse the prognosis is.
  - Muscle rigidity, trismus, autonomic failure, rhabdomyolysis, and death occur in 15%–30% of cases.
  - Treatment consists of human tetanus immunoglobulin, diazepam, or baclofen and supportive care. Debridement of the infected wound source is crucial.

CASE 20.1B: RESOLUTION WITH BACLOFEN PUMP

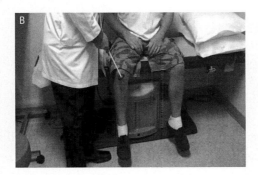

VIDEO 20.1B

The patient was treated with intrathecal baclofen. Within a day, the spasms resolved and he was able to walk without a cane, and tapping the patellar tendon did not produce cramping.

Deep tendon reflexes are absent due to baclofen.

CASE 20.2: CARPAL SPASMS

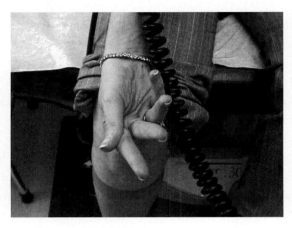

VIDEO 20.2

A 27-year-old woman presented with recurrent painful spasms of the hands and feet muscles. She had several panic attacks after the recent death of her mother.

The demonstrated signs are:

1. Trousseau sign
2. Babinski sign
3. Chvostek sign
4. Oppenheim sign
5. Chaddock sign

DIAGNOSIS

- Tetany is peripheral nerves hyperexcitability due to acute hypocalcemia. Low serum calcium enhances sodium influx to the cells and thus triggers depolarization.
- The most clinical features of hypocalcemia are:
  - Perioral and acral paresthesias
  - Carpopedal spasms: flexion of the writs and metacarpophalangeal joints (MPJs) and extension of the interphalangeal joints (IPJs)
  - Stiffness, myalgia, clumsiness, and fatigue
  - Trousseau sign: inflation of sphygmomanometer above systolic blood pressure (BP) for 3 minutes leads to carpal spasms due to increased excitability of the nerve trunks by ischemia. Hyperexcitability peaks in 3 minutes and returns to normal afterward, even if ischemia continues.
  - Chovstek sign: tapping the facial nerve leads to contraction of the ipsilateral facial muscles. It occurs in 10% of normal people.
  - Laryngeal strider
  - Seizures
  - Cardiac involvement: prolonged Q-T interval, hypotension, and arrhythmias
- EMG: repeated high frequency discharges after a single stimulation is typical. Doublet and triplet fasciculations are common.
- Hyperventilation leads to respiratory alkalosis, which causes conversion of ionized calcium to protein bound calcium. Despite preservation of the total serum calcium concentration, the drop in the ionized, physiologically active, calcium leads to tetany.
- Other causes of hypocalcemia include chronic renal failure, malabsorption syndrome, hypoparathyroidism, and hypomagnesaemia.
- Treatment of hyperventilation is by reassurance and treatment of the underlying anxiety.
- Rebreathing from a plastic bag has not been tested systematically and may cause hypoxia and therefore cannot be recommended.

CASE 20.3: CRAMPING AND HYPERTROPHY OF THE CALVES

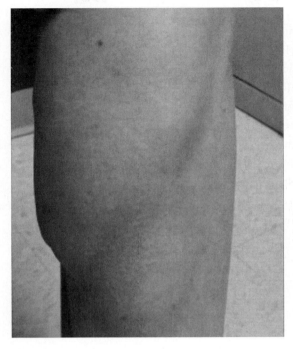

VIDEO 20.3

A 44-year-old woman presented with diffuse muscle pain and episodic painful cramping of the calf muscles for a 1-year duration. CPK level was 420U/L, and EMG revealed high frequency (120 Hz) discharges.

The following can cause enlargement of the calves:

1. Amyloidosis
2. Hypothyroidism
3. Neuromyotonia
4. Dysferlinopathy
5. Facioscapulohumeral muscular dystrophy (FSHD)

DIAGNOSIS

Calves hypertrophy may be caused by:

- Deposition of non-muscle tissue:
  - Such as amyloid (amyloidosis)
  - Mucopolysaccharides (hypothyroidism)
  - Fatty tissue (Duchenne muscular dystrophy)
- Hypertrophy of muscles due to hyperactivity:
  - Peripheral nerve hyperexcitability such as neuromyotonia
  - Chronic neurogenic insults such as some cases of chronic inflammatory demyelinating polyneuropathy (CIDP) and S1 radiculopathy
- Ultrasound helps differentiate these two categories.
- EMG shows decreased insertional activity in the first category.
- Dysferlinopathy typically causes calf atrophy.

CASE 20.4A: STIFF BACK MUSCLES

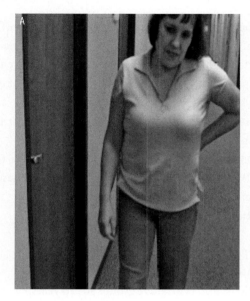

VIDEO 20.4A

A 43-year-old woman presented with intermittent painful cramping of the back muscles starting 3 years earlier. The spasms increased in frequency and severity to a degree that she could not work any more. She had normal strength and deep tendon reflexes (DTRs). CPK was normal and EMG revealed continuous discharges of motor unit potential (MUP) of normal configuration and frequency. She responded well to diazepam up to 40 mg a day with no sleepiness.

What test is likely to be abnormal?

1. GAD antibodies
2. VGKC antibodies
3. S. Ca level
4. S. Mg level
5. Spastin mutation analysis

DIAGNOSIS

- Stiff person syndrome is an autoimmune disorder caused by antibodies against glutamic acid decarboxylase. These antibodies localize to GABAnergic neurons.
- GABA is an important inhibitory neurotransmitter, and its absence causes spasticity.
- GAD also targets pancreatic beta cells, which explains the increased incidence (25% of cases) of DM type 1 in these patients.
- GAD antibodies are positive in 60% of cases and the CSF GAD antibodies are more specific than the serum GAD antibodies.
- 70% of DM-I patients have positive GAD antibodies, but the titer is usually less than 10-fold, while in SPS it is usually 100–500-fold. In addition, these antibodies recognized deferent epitopes of GAD.
- There are three variants of SPS:
  - Autoimmune
  - Paraneoplastic
  - Idiopathic: negative serology, 30%
- Female to male ratio is: 3:1. Typical age group: 30–70 years.
- Muscle stiffness and rigidity start in the axial muscles leading to spinal grooving.
- Severe intermittent spasms can be crippling.
- Paroxysmal dysautonomia (hyperpyrexia diaphoresis, tachycardia, mydriasis, and hypertension) may result in sudden death.
- Most people respond to diazepam. Sometimes, doses as high as 100 mg a day are needed.
- Interestingly, sleepiness is not a common side effect in patients with SPS.
- Immunomodulation with azathioprine, IVIG, and plasmapheresis are other options in refractory cases.
- 64% of patients remain ambulatory with extended follow-up (up to 23 years).

CASE 20.4B: STIFF PERSON SYNDROME
AFTER TREATMENT

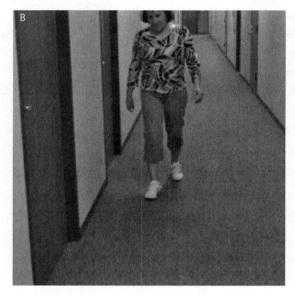

VIDEO 20.4B

DIAGNOSIS

- Diazepam as a GABA agonist is the drug of choice to which most patients respond at least early in the course of the disease.
- The starting dose is 5 mg TID with gradual titration. Cases are reported to have needed 300 mg a day for symptoms control.
- Oral or intravenous (IV) baclofen is also effective in severe cases.
- IV solumedrol, IV gammaglobulin are shown to be effective in refractory cases.
- Plasmapheresis and Rituximab are other options.
- Some patients become refractory after an initial response to diazepam.
- GAD antibody titer does not correlate with severity or improvement.

CASE 20.5: INABILITY TO ROLL OVER IN BED

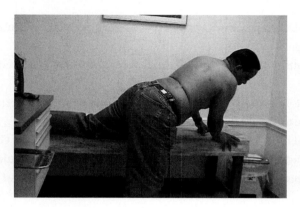

VIDEO 20.5

A 41-year-old man presented with gradually worsening and disabling stiffness of the back muscles as shown in the video. He had intermittent stiffness of the legs muscles, worsened by stress. Examination revealed normal deep tendon reflexes and strength and normal CK level. GAD Ab titer was 70 times the upper limit of normal.

GAD-65 antibodies are reported in 80% of DM type 1, yet SPS is rare. This is explainable by the fact that:

1. These GAD antibodies recognize different epitopes of the enzyme.
2. Many diabetics have subclinical SPS.
3. GAD antibodies are not pathogenic.
4. The studies that produced these results are not consistent.
5. SPS is genetic.

DIAGNOSIS

- 70%–80% of DM type 1 cases are associated with elevated GAD antibodies, yet SPS is a rare disease.
- The GAD antibody titer is much higher in SPS than observed in DM 1 (up to 1,000-fold).
- Sera from SPS but non-diabetic patients recognize a linear NH2 terminal epitope residing within the first eight amino acids of GAD.
- Sera from DM type-1 patients recognize conformational epitope of GAD.
- T-cells respond to different epitopes: two regions of GAD molecules produced T-cells proliferative responses in 6 of 8 patients with SPS, but in only 1 out of 17 with type 1 DM.

REFERENCES

Kim J, et al. Higher autoantibody levels and recognition of a linear NH2-terminal epitope in the autoantigen GAD65, distinguish stiff-man syndrome from insulin-dependent diabetes mellitus. *J Exp Med*. 1994;180(2):595.

Lohmann T, et al. Immune reactivity to glutamic acid decarboxylase 65 in stiffman syndrome and type 1 diabetes mellitus. *Lancet*. 2000;356(9223):31.

CASE 20.6: MUSCLE CRAMPS AND DIARRHEA

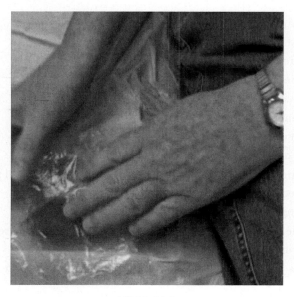

VIDEO 20.6

A 55-year-old woman presented with a several-year history of severe intermittent painful spasms of the arm and leg muscles lasting minutes to hours and occurring many times a day. Stool examination showed high fat contents. She had no muscle weakness. She had a history of hypothyroidism.

This combination of symptoms suggests:

1. Gluten enteropathy
2. Alopecia universalis
3. Satayoshi syndrome
4. Neuromyotonia
5. Hyperthyroidism

DIAGNOSIS

- Satayoshi syndrome is a triad of diarrhea, alopecia, and muscle cramps.
- It is a multisystemic disease presumed to be autoimmune in nature.
- Adolescents are the main target, but adult onset cases are reported.
- It is more common in females.
- The immune nature is supported by:
  - Improvement with steroids
  - Association with other immune diseases
  - Deposition of immune complexes in the muscles
- The spasms can be very severe and progressive, leading to abnormal posturing and problems with speech.
- Malabsorption may lead to nutritional deficiency.
- Sclerosis of the growth plate due to recurrent trauma produced by severe muscle spasms is characteristic.
- Severe spasms may respond to dantrolene, and calcium gluconate or even botulinum toxin.
- The disease usually responds to steroids or IVIG.

REFERENCE

Asherson RA, et al. A case of adult-onset Satoyoshi syndrome with gastric ulceration and eosinophilic enteritis. *Nat Clin Pract Rheumatol.* 2008 Aug;4(8):439–444.

CASE 20.7: MUSCLE CRAMPS AFTER BARIATRIC SURGERY

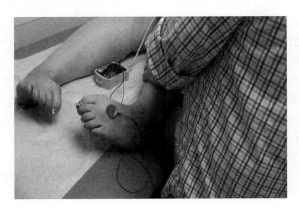

VIDEO 20.7

A 31-year-old woman had developed muscle cramps 3 years after gastric bypass surgery that resulted in a 150-pound weight loss. The cramps were severe enough to dislocate a hip joint and twist her feet violently. She became disabled. She could not tolerate an EMG, and her CK level was 340 U/L. She was taking multivitamins and calcium 500 mg a day since surgery. Serum calcium was 5.6 mg/dl (normal 8.5–10.5), alkaline phosphatase was 500 U/L (20–120). Phosphorus and magnesium levels were normal. She had macrocytic anemia.

Complications of gastric bypass surgery:

1. Severe muscle cramps
2. Hypocalcemia
3. Polyneuropathy
4. Myopathy
5. Copper deficiency

DIAGNOSIS

- Gastric bypass surgery has become one of the most common surgeries in modern times.
- There are many types of bariatric surgery; all of them are associated with neuromuscular complications, although gastric sleeves have a more benign course.
- Complications can be immediate or remote and may occur up to 20 years after surgery.
- Commonly reported neuromuscular complications are:
  - Peripheral neuropathy:
    - Polyneuropathy, including Guillain-Barré syndrome
    - Mononeuropathy, including meralgia paresthetica
  - Myopathy and rhabdomyolysis: myalgia is common in hypocalcemia due to pseudofractures
  - Lumbar plexitis
  - Myeloneuropathy: typically seen in copper deficiency
- The causes of these complications are not clear.
  - An inflammatory basis has been suggested
  - Deficiency of vitamins, minerals, and micronutrients (selenium, cadmium, etc.)
- Monitoring of micronutrients level and prompt recognition can reduce morbidity.
- Most neuromuscular complications are remote and gradually evolving.
- Copper deficiency usually occurs after years and presents with sensory ataxia and hyper-reflexia due to myeloneuropathy.
- Hypocalcemia due to Vitamin D deficiency is the most common cause of muscle cramps. Up to 30% of patients develop hypocalcemia.
- Correction of hypocalcemia effectively improves myalgia and muscle cramps in many patients.

CASE 20.8: LEFT LEG STIFFNESS AND FALLS

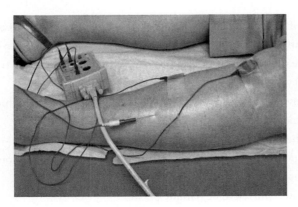

VIDEO 20.8

A 77-year-old woman presented with a 1-year history of intermittent spasms of the left leg muscles with occasional inversion of the foot, leading to falls. She has a history of right S1 radiculopathy. Electromogram is shown.

Which test is most appropriate?

1. AChR antibody titer
2. GAD antibody titer
3. VGKC antibody titer
4. SCN4 mutation
5. VGCC antibody titer

DIAGNOSIS

- The stiffness of the left leg and continuous EMG activity suggested stiff person syndrome (SPS). GAD antibody level was 100 nmol/L. Focal SPS is difficult to diagnose.
- Focal SPS usually starts in a leg (stiff leg syndrome) and spares the trunk.
- Onset: 35–60 years
- Stiffness is provoked by voluntary movement and sensory stimuli, which may cause severe stiffness and torsion of the feet and falls.
- GAD antibodies level does not correlate with severity.
- It usually responds partially to diazepam and baclofen. Intravenous immunoglobulin (IVIG) may lead to temporary improvement.
- Focal SPS is not reported to be paraneoplastic.
- Since isolated leg stiffness is the most common symptom, serologic confirmation is important for the diagnosis.
- It is possible that many seronegative cases are missed.
- In some cases, stiffness generalizes within 2 years, but most cases remain restricted.

REFERENCES

Meinck HM, et al. Stiff man syndrome and related conditions. *Move Dis.* 2002 Sep;17(5):853–866.

McKeon A, et al. Stiff-man syndrome and variants clinical course, treatments, and outcomes *Arch Neurol.* 2012;69(2):230–238.

CASE 20.9: STIFFNESS AND HYPERTROPHY OF THE THENAR MUSCLES

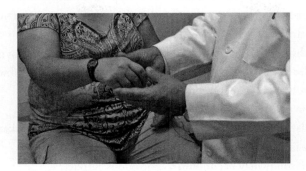

VIDEO 20.9

A 41-year-old woman presented with a several-year history of intermittent muscle cramps involving the hands and sweating. Gradually, the small hand muscles, especially the thenar muscles, became hypertrophic and contracted most of the time but were not weak. The EMG is shown.

Which test is most appropriate?

1. AChR Abs
2. GAD Abs
3. VGKC Abs
4. SCN4 mutation
5. VGCC Abs

DIAGNOSIS

- Neuromyotonia is a form of peripheral nerve hyperexcitability where there are spontaneous irregular bursts of single motor unit potentials at a frequency of 40–300 Hz.
- Age: 9–80 years
- Muscle twitching, stiffness, and cramping are the main presenting symptoms.
- Distal muscles are affected more than proximal muscles, and stiffness is worsened by exercises leading to diagnostic confusion with paramyotonia.
- No percussion myotonia is noted.
- Activity persists during sleep but is blocked by neuromuscular blockers.
- Usually there is no associated weakness of the affected muscles.
- Muscle hypertrophy may occur due to continuous activity.
- No spontaneous remission usually occurs, but fluctuation is common.
- Thymoma, lymphoma, and lung cancer are the most frequently associated neoplasms.
- CK level is elevated in 50% of cases.
- VGKC antibodies are increased in two-thirds of cases.
- Carbamazepine and mexiletine usually help the cramps.
- Steroids and IVIG usually lead to short-term benefit.
- Clinical syndromes with VGKC antibodies:
  - Neuromyotonia
  - Myokymia
  - Cramp fasciculation syndrome
  - Benign fasciculation syndrome
  - Morvan syndrome
  - Limbic encephalitis
  - Painful polyneuropathy

CASE 20.10: SILENT MUSCLE CRAMPS

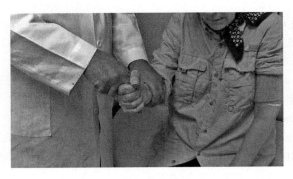

VIDEO 20.10

A 62-year-old woman presented with muscle cramps since childhood. Gradually, the cramps became severe and generalized and were associated with poor relaxation of the contracted muscles. She had mild proximal weakness and the CK was normal. EMG of the cramping muscles was silent.

The most important causes of electrically silent muscle cramps are:

1. McArdle disease
2. Paramyotonia
3. Brody disease
4. Neuromyotonia
5. Stiff person syndrome (SPS)

DIAGNOSIS

- Brody disease is a rare disorder characterized by impaired skeletal muscle contraction following exercises.
- Activity-induced cramping and stiffness.
- Rapid closure and opening of the fists or eyelids may lead to delayed relaxation.
- There is no percussion myotonia.
- CK level is usually normal.
- EMG usually shows that the muscles that fail to relax are electrically silent, similar to what happens in McArdle disease, but there is a normal rise of serum lactate and ammonia during forearm ischemic exercise test.
- Muscle biopsy shows Type 2 fiber atrophy and reduced Ca-ATPase in type 2 muscle fibers with immunohistochemistry staining.
- It is caused by an autosomal recessive mutation of ATPA1 gene or autosomal dominant with normal ATPA1 gene.
- This gene encodes sarcoplasmic reticulum calcium-ATPase (SERCA1), a calcium channel present on the SR of type 2 fibers.
- Dantrolene is usually effective.

CASE 20.11: MUSCLE CRAMPS AND FEET NUMBNESS

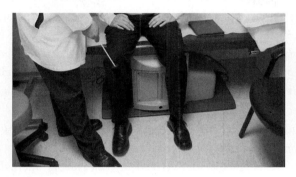

VIDEO 20.11

A 53-year-old man presented with a long history of smoking and daily alcohol drinking who developed painful spasms of the calves, feet numbness, and poor balance over 3 months. Nerve conduction study (NCS) revealed mild axonal neuropathy. B_{12} level was 250 pg/ml. Examination is shown in the video.

The next appropriate step is:

1. Magnetic resonance imaging (MRI) cervical spines
2. Lumbar spine magnetic resonance imaging (LS MRI)
3. Treat B_{12} deficiency
4. Chest computed tomography (CT) scan
5. Cerebrospinal fluid (CSF) examination

DIAGNOSIS

- Sustained painful muscle spasms can be produced by increased muscle tone due to upper motor neurons lesions such as myelopathies, hereditary spastic paraplegia, tropical spastic paraplegia, and amyotrophic lateral sclerosis (ALS).
- The sustained spasms are due to loss of central inhibition of the lower motor neurons.
- Although the patient had axonal neuropathy, most likely alcohol related, this finding is minor compared to the gait spasticity and hyperreflexia and neurogenic bladder, and it should not preclude further investigations.
- Spinal tap should be avoided before a compressive lesion is ruled out due to possible worsening of the compression after spinal tap.
- Borderline B_{12} level should be verified by measuring methylmalonic acid and homocysteine.
- While myelopathy and neuropathy are features of B_{12} deficiency, sensory ataxia is much more pronounced than spasticity in these cases.
- History of smoking suggests lung cancer, which can cause cord compression or paraneoplastic neuropathy.
- Involvement of the arms and legs with upper motor neuron (UMN) signs suggest cervical myelopathy. Structural lesions are the most common, in particular cervical spondylosis, HNP, and tumors.
- The rest of the possibilities mentioned above should be investigated and treated as well.
- The most appropriate next step therefore, is to obtain a cervical spines MRI.

CHAPTER 21

MYOTONIA

CASE 21.1: A FAMILY WITH MUSCLE STIFFNESS

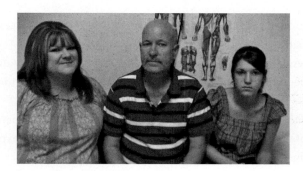

VIDEO 21.1

A 53-year-old man had noticed difficulty relaxing his hand grip after a handshake at age 35 years. Gradually he developed stiffness of the leg muscles and cataracts. His asymptomatic daughter's examination revealed grip and percussion myotonia.

The earlier appearance of symptoms in the daughter is due to a phenomenon called:

1. Contraction
2. Anticipation
3. Variable penetrance
4. Heteroplasmy
5. Co-dominance

DIAGNOSIS

- The phenomenon of earlier onset and more severe symptoms in successive generations is called "anticipation."
- This is an interesting genetic phenomenon that was thought to be due to a bias resulting from more attention being given to the disease-related symptoms in the younger generation.
- It is clear now that this phenomenon is due to the instability of a genetic mutation.
- It is mostly noted in genetic disorders that are characterized by the expansion of trinucleotide repeats beyond a threshold.
- Triple repeats exist in human genomes coding and non-coding components; most of the time, their expansion is harmless.
- Examples of diseases caused by trinucleotide repeat expansion:
  - Myotonic dystrophy type 1 (DM 1)
  - Huntington disease
  - Fragile X syndrome
  - Machado-Joseph disease
  - Friedreich ataxia
- In myotonic dystrophy type 1, the expanded repeat is a CTG sequence in the non-coding region of protein kinase gene on chromosome 19.
  - A normal CTG repeat number is between 5 and 37.
  - A range of 38–49 repeats is called permutation range, and it increases the risk of having affected children.
  - A repeat of more than 50 is almost always symptomatic.
  - Interestingly, the number of CTG repeats positively correlates with an earlier onset and more severe disease.
  - The expanded repeats tend to expand further during meiosis leading to a larger repeat in successive generations which explains the phenomenon of anticipation.
  - The cause of instability of the CTG repeat is not clear.
  - More interestingly, CTG repeats expand when they go through a female germline and only rarely through a male germline. This explains the congenital form of the disease.

REFERENCE

Athni S, Shaibani A, Ashizawa T. Anticipation and myotonic dystrophy: Diagnostic and prognostic implications. *Resident and Staff Physician*. 1996;42:57–63.

CASE 21.2: MYALGIA AND MYOTONIA

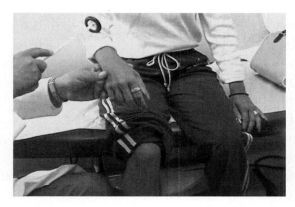

VIDEO 21.2

A 36-year-old woman presented with severe painful spasms of the lower back muscles for 3 years that gradually worsened and spread to the chest muscles, hands, and feet. She did not respond to baclofen, topiramate, and hydromorphone. She became disabled. Her neurologists found diffuse myotonic discharges in the electromyogram (EMG) and therefore referred her for consultation. Mutation analysis revealed no CTG repeat expansion on chromosome 19.

The most appropriate next test is to look for mutation(s) in the following gene(s):

1. Sodium channel
2. Chloride channel
3. Zinc finger protein 9 (ZNF9)
4. Potassium channel
5. Mitochondria

DIAGNOSIS

- Myotonic dystrophy type 2 is caused by mutation of zinc finger protein 9 (ZNF9) on chromosome 3q21.
- The phenomenon of anticipation is much less common than DM type 1.
- Congenital form is rare.
- Weakness is more proximal than distal.
- Face is affected in only 12% of cases.
- Calves hypertrophy is reported.
- Myalgia and stiffness occur in 56% of cases and are:
  - Induced by sensory stimuli and palpation or percussion of the affected muscles
  - Increase with cold
  - Not related to severity of myotonia
  - Affect proximal (including chest) more than distal muscles, leading to suspicion of coronary heart disease, which is enforced by creatine kinase (CK) elevation
- Central nervous system (CNS) involvement is rare.
- Systemic manifestations:
  - Cataracts: 100% over 20 years as visualized with slit lamp examination
  - Cardiac arrhythmias: 20%; conduction defects
  - Diabetes mellitus: 20%
  - Hearing loss: 20%
  - Fertility: normal or reduced
  - Cardiovascular autonomic function: normal
- More benign course than myotonic dystrophy type 1.

REFERENCE

http://neuromuscular.wustl.edu/

CASE 21.3: HAND NUMBNESS AND DIFFUSE ABNORMAL DISCHARGES

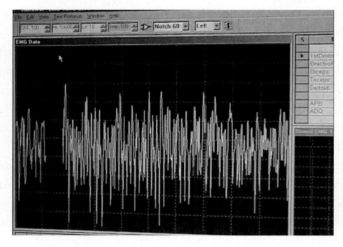

VIDEO 21.3

A 35-year-old woman visited a neurologist for hand numbness. EMG revealed the displayed discharges in many tested muscles in the arms and legs. She also had a mild prolongation of the palmar median sensory latency bilaterally that explained her hand numbness.

These discharges can be seen in the following disorders:

1. Myotonia congenita
2. Schwartz Jampel syndrome
3. Myotonic dystrophy
4. Brody syndrome
5. McArdle disease

DIAGNOSIS

- Myotonia is a slow relaxation of skeletal muscles after contraction.
- Muscle fibers are hyperexcitable and they repetitively discharge after a contraction, which results in slow relaxation.
- The contraction is purely myogenic, regardless of the motor neuron activity.
- These discharges may be provoked by voluntary contraction (action myotonia), mechanical tapping (percussion myotonia), or needle insertion (electromechanical myotonia).
- Electrically, they appear as waxing and waning positive discharges (fibrillations and positive sharp waves) in a frequency of 20–80 Hz, similar to accelerating and decelerating motorcycle engine.
- Sometimes patients are referred to neuromuscular clinics because these discharges are discovered during an EMG that is done for a related (stiffness, weakness, etc.) or non-related (hand numbness) cause.
- These discharges may be confused with diffuse denervation (e.g., motor neuron disease), neuromyotonia (faster discharges than 150 Hz), or complex repetitive discharges (end abruptly and do not wax and wane).
- Subclinical myotonia is usually a feature of chloride channelopathy and to a lesser extent Na channelopathy.
- Resting electrical features do not practically distinguish among different myotonic disorders, but short exercise test often does.
- There are disorders that are characterized by muscle stiffness and cramping that sometimes are confused clinically as myotonic disorders, but the EMG is silent. Examples are Brody syndrome and McArdle disease.
- Causes of myotonia include:
  - Myotonic dystrophy
  - Non-dystrophic myotonia (chloride and Na channelopathies)
  - Metabolic myopathies such as acid maltase deficiency
  - Toxic myopathies such as statin myopathy
  - Endocrine myopathy such as hypothyroidism
  - Inflammatory myopathies
  - Myofibrillar myopathies
  - Schwartz Jampel syndrome

CASE 21.4: PERSISTENT HAND SHAKING

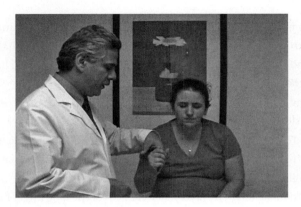

VIDEO 21.4

A 32-year-old woman presented with stiffness of the hand muscles during winter.
Hand shaking is often diagnostically useful in:

1. Inclusion body myositis
2. Duchenne muscular dystrophy
3. Myotonic dystrophy
4. Acid maltase deficiency
5. Mitochondrial myopathy

DIAGNOSIS

- Hand shaking is one of the diagnostic tools in the neuromuscular clinic.
- Parents' advice to their children to look at a person's face while shaking hands applies to the neuromuscular examination as well. The face, along with the hand, is very often a source of diagnostic information.
- Myotonic hand contracts normally but relaxes slowly. A forceful contraction is usually followed by a slow relaxation.
- Repeated hand shaking leads to improvement of myotonia (warming up phenomenon) in myotonic dystrophy and chloride channelopathies (myotonia congenita) and worsening of myotonia in Na channelopathy (paramyotonia congenita).
- In patients with inclusion body myositis, weakness of the long finger flexors and preservation of the finger extensors and intrinsic hands muscles lead to a "fish mouth hand" during shaking, as the fingers cannot be flexed at the interphalangeal joint.
- While myotonic discharges are reported in acid maltase deficiency, it mostly occurs in thoracic paraspinal muscles and not in the distal muscles.
- Duchenne muscular dystrophy and mitochondrial myopathy do not have special hand features.

CASE 21.5: FAMILIAL SENSITIVITY TO COLD

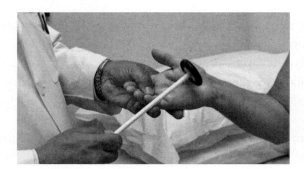

VIDEO 21.5

A 55-year-old woman had moved from Chicago to Houston due to cold-induced muscle stiffness. Her mother had a similar problem. She saw a neurologist in Houston for neck pain radiating to the right arm and he found her to have diffuse waxing and waning 100 Hz discharges in several tested muscles. There was no mutation in the sodium channel (SCN4) gene.

The most appropriate next test is to look for:

1. CTG repeat expansion at the DMPK gene
2. Chloride channel (CLCN1) gene mutation
3. Calcium channel gene mutation
4. Voltage gated potassium channel mutation
5. None of the above

Unlike paramyotonia congenita, myotonia congenita is usually:

1. An always autosomal dominant disorder
2. Often cold sensitive
3. It warms up with repetition
4. It does not show decremental response
5. Is associated with hyperkalemic periodic paralysis

DIAGNOSIS

- The most important question when myotonia is clinically or electrically found is whether this is a dystrophic or non-dystrophic myotonia (NDM).
  - The phenotype of myotonic dystrophy is characteristic (thin and weak face, temporal wasting, cataract, mental dullness, distal and proximal weakness). Myotonic dystrophy, especially type 2, may present with only myotonia and pain, leading to diagnostic difficulty.
  - It is has been observed that NDM patients sometimes have rounded faces due to occasional hypertrophy of temporalis muscles from myotonic discharges.
- The second question is whether NDM is due to chloride (myotonia congenita) or Na channelopathy (paramyotonia congenita).
  - Myotonia congenita (MC) is usually a chloride channelopathy and may be recessive or dominant, while paramyotonia congenita (PMC) is usually due to Na channelopathy and it is allelic to hyperkalemic periodic paralysis (HYPP). It is an autosomal dominant disorder.
  - Extreme sensitivity to cold is mostly seen in PMC and is rare in MC.
  - Warming up after repetitive testing is a feature of MC. PMC gets worse with repetition (paradoxical myotonia).
  - Episodic weakness and lid myotonia are see in PMC but rarely in MC.
  - Warming up and sensitivity to cold can be confirmed neurophysiologically by a long exercise test.
  - Both decrement with 2 Hz repetitive nerve stimulation test. Cooling increased decrement in PMC.
  - Myotonia caused by CLCN1 mutations can occasionally be clinically indistinguishable from myotonia caused by sodium channel mutations (SCN4A mutations) resulting in paramyotonia congenita (PMC).

REFERENCES

Matthews E, et al. The non-dystrophic myotonias: molecular pathogenesis, diagnosis and treatment. *Brain*. 2010 Jan;133(1):9–22.

Michel P, et al. Comparative efficacy of repetitive nerve simulation, exercise, and cold in differentiating myotonic disorders. *Muscle and Nerve*. 2007;36(5):643–650.

CASE 21.6: STIFFNESS THAT GETS BETTER WITH USE

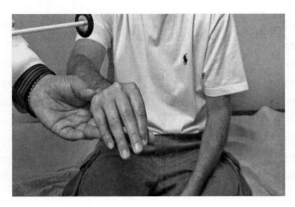

VIDEO 21.6

A 47-year-old man presented with muscle stiffness that started at age 21 years. His parents had premature cataracts and his sister and three maternal aunts were diagnosed with myotonic dystrophy based on the presence of CTG repeat expansion on chromosome 19.

The demonstrated phenomenon is a cardinal feature of:

1. Sodium channelopathies
2. Chloride channelopathies
3. Calcium channelopathies
4. Myotonic dystrophy
5. Potassium channelopathies

DIAGNOSIS

- The most common sites of demonstrating myotonia clinically are wrists extensors, thenar muscles, tongue, and eyelids.
  - Tapping wrist extensors leads to slow return of the extended wrist to the baseline.
  - Tapping thenar muscles leads to slow return of the thumb to its position.
  - Excreting pressure on the tongue leads to grooving due to slow relaxation of the tapped muscles.
  - Lid myotonia is seen more commonly in PMC (also it is seen in hypokalemic periodic paralysis). It is easy to demonstrate paradoxical myotonia by asking the patient to close eyes repeatedly. With more closure, eye opening becomes more difficult and the eyelids stick to each other longer.
- **Warm up phenomenon** was initially reported in MC patients as they get stiffer in the morning and after a long rest, and their muscle stiffness eases up with exercise and daily muscle use.
- Patients with myotonic dystrophy demonstrate the same phenomenon.
- The molecular biology of this phenomenon is not clear. Mild slowing of Na channel inactivation is thought to be the cause.

REFERENCE

Lossin C. Nav1.4 slow-inactivation: is it a player in the warm-up phenomenon of myotonic disorders? *Muscle & Nerve*. 2013;47(4):483–487.

CASE 21.7: STIFFNESS WORSENED BY ANXIETY

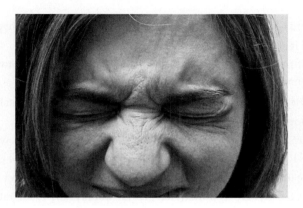

VIDEO 21.7

A 34-year-old woman presented with muscle stiffness worsened by cold temperature and stress.

The demonstrated sign can be seen in:

1. Paramyotonia congenita (PMC)
2. Myotonia congenita (MC)
3. Hypokalemic periodic paralysis (HypoKPP)
4. Polymyositis
5. Oculopharyngeal muscular dystrophy

DIAGNOSIS

- Eyelid myotonia is a feature of PMC and is sometimes observed in hypokalemic periodic paralysis, but it is not a feature of myotonia congenita.
- Worsening of myotonia with repetitive motion (paradoxical myotonia) is a feature of PMC.
- Cold sensitivity is also an important feature of the disease and can be demonstrated neurophysiologically.
- PMC is an autosomal dominant mutation of sodium channels Alpha subunit (SCN4A) on chromosome 17q23.3. Rarely paramyotonia is produced by chloride channel mutation.
- PMC is allelic to hyperkalemic periodic paralysis, and they can affect the same patient.
- Mutated Na channels are dysfunctional and are abnormally inactivated, leading to continuous leak of Na into cell.
- Symptoms usually appear in the first decade of life. During a crying episode, infants may have difficulty opening their eyes due to "exercise induced" myotonia.
- Weakness is not prominent, and CK is usually normal or slightly high.
- Mexiletine 150–1,000 mg/day is shown to be effective in a double blind trial.

REFERENCE

Statland JM, et al. Mexiletine for symptoms and signs of myotonia in non-dystrophic myotonia. *JAMA.* 2012;308(13):1357–1365.

CASE 21.8: EPISODIC WEAKNESS AND MUSCLE STIFFNESS

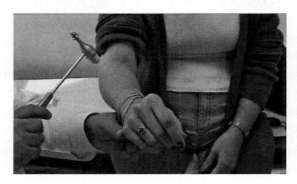

VIDEO 21.8

A 35-year-old woman had developed an episode of paralysis lasting hours after hearing about her father's death at age 15. Since then she had milder episodic morning weakness that improves after eating cereal for breakfast. Her examination was shown in the video.

This condition is typically associated with:

1. SCN4A mutation
2. Paramyotonia congenita (PMC)
3. Hyperkalemic periodic paralysis
4. Myotonic dystrophy
5. Myotonia congenita (MC)

DIAGNOSIS

- The examination shows myotonia that gets worse with repetitive testing (paradoxical myotonia). This is typically seen in paramyotonia congenita (PMC).
- Recurrent episodic weakness (periodic paralysis) may be familial or non-familial (thyrotoxic, hypokalemic, etc.).
- Familial periodic paralysis could be potassium sensitive (hyperkalemic) or hypokalemic.
- Hyperkalemic periodic paralysis may present without myotonia, with myotonia, or is associated with a full-blown PMC.
- Cooling usually triggers attacks when PMC is present.
- Myotonia is usually subtle and can be elicited by percussing the thenar eminence, fingers extensors, and pressing the tongue.
- The attacks usually start in the first decade and occur in the mornings, triggered by rest after exercise, ingestion of potassium-rich food, fasting, and stress.
- Degree of weakness varies, and weakness usually starts in the legs.
- The sphincters, bulbar, and respiratory muscles are usually preserved.
- Frequency of attacks greatly varies from several times a day to once a year; each usually lasts less than 2 hours, and they are rarely profound.
- During the attacks, deep tendon reflexes are usually absent. Between the attacks, eyelid myotonia may be the only finding.
- Creatine kinase may be slightly elevated and serum potassium is usually normal, but urinary excretion of potassium is high.
- If serum potassium is high, one has to rule out other causes of hyperkalemia.
- Treatment with intravenous (IV) glucose and insulin is only needed in severe attacks. Mild attacks resolve spontaneously.
- Acetazolamide and chlorothiazide may reduce the frequency of attacks.

CASE 21.9: MUSCLE STIFFNESS AND ABORTIONS

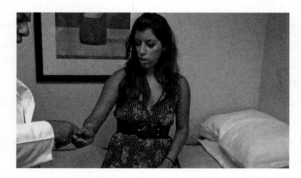

VIDEO 21.9

A 27-year-old woman presented with a 7-year history of muscle stiffness and "failure of relaxation of contracted muscles." Her mother was wheelchair bound due to leg weakness, and she had a sister with dropped head and leg weakness. The patient had two abortions.

The following is (are) true about the genetics of this condition:

1. Anticipation is associated with longer CTG repeat.
2. CTG repeats occur in the coding region of the DMPK gene.
3. Variable penetrance is a common feature.
4. Permutations are associated with severe disease.
5. Congenital cases occur equally through father's and mother's lines.

DIAGNOSIS

- Myotonic dystrophy (DM) is the most prevalent neuromuscular disorder in adults.
- 98% of cases are type 1 (DM1). Females and males have equal chances of being affected.
- Penetrance is variable, but it is 100% by age 50 years.
- It is a multisystemic disease. Systemic features include cataract, cardiac conduction abnormalities, diabetes mellitus, hypothyroidism, cognitive abnormalities, and GI motility disorder.
- The disease is cause by a CTG repeat expansion in the non-coding region of dystrophia myotonica protein kinase (DMPK).
- Clinical severity correlates with the size of repeat expansion.
- The mutation is unstable, and the appearance of the disease at an earlier age and in a more severe form in subsequent generations (anticipation) is due to expansion of the CTG repeat during meiosis.
- The repeat size is greater in muscle than blood cells, but it does not correlate with muscle weakness.
- Myotonia is more common in younger age groups, while weakness is more common in older population.
- Weakness of finger flexors and face and dysphagia may be confused with inclusion body myositis (IBM).
- Annual electrocardiogram (ECG) to detect conduction abnormalities is recommended.
- Sudden death is mostly due to cardiac arrhythmias or respiratory failure. Tricyclic antidepressants, digoxin, procainamide, propranolol, and Quinine are to be avoided.
- If a patient decides to become pregnant, prenatal diagnosis is possible. A high-risk perinatal care is recommended.
- The disease is not curable. Progress has been made in animal models to reduce the toxic gain of function that is created by the expanded repeats. Charles Thornton's group used antisense oligonucleotides to target mutant RNA that is retained in the nucleus and exerts a toxic gain of function. They reported correction of physiological and histopathologic features that sustained for up to a year after treatment was discontinued.

REFERENCE

Wheeler TM, et al. Targeting nuclear RNA for in vivo correction of myotonic dystrophy. *Nature*. 2012 Aug 2;488(7409):111–115.

CASE 21.10: ASYMPTOMATIC PARAMYOTONIA CONGENITA

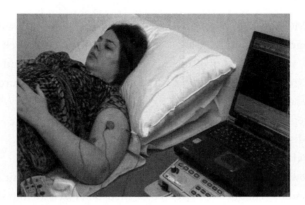

VIDEO 21.10

A 28-year-old woman from Houston was referred by a rheumatologist who found diffuse abnormal discharges during EMG while evaluating her arm numbness. She did not give history of weakness. She had two vague episodes of muscle stiffness during childhood when she visited her father in Minnesota. Her examination revealed normal strength. Amplitude of compound muscle action potential of the thenar muscles decreased after exercise.

The following diagnostic test(s) is (are) appropriate:

1. Sodium channel mutation analysis
2. Chloride channel mutation analysis
3. Resting serum potassium concentration
4. Calcium channels mutation analysis
5. Muscle biopsy

The following is (are) true about this condition:

1. It is an X-linked recessive disease.
2. Cold exposure increases post-exercise decremental response.
3. It is often associated with cardiac involvement.
4. It is associated with hyperkalemic periodic paralysis.
5. It is frequently asymptomatic.

DIAGNOSIS

- The lack of EMG findings to explain clinical abnormalities such as weakness, muscle atrophy, or numbness is a common cause of referrals to neuromuscular clinics.
- Nevertheless, unexplained or incidental EMG abnormalities found in general neurology practice are, although less frequently, an equally important source of such referrals. Examples of these findings:
  - Complex repetitive discharges confused with myotonic discharges
  - Myotonic discharges confused with diffuse denervation
  - Positive sharp waves disease
- The video shows percussion thenar myotonia and electrical myotonic discharges.
- Mutation of sodium channel SCN4A is confirmed. SCN4A is an important cause of myotonia and is found in patients with paramyotonia congenita and hyperkalemic periodic paralysis and in 10% of patients with hypokalemic periodic paralysis.
- Chloride channel mutations are usually asymptomatic and can be inherited as autosomal dominant or recessive. Myotonia is not as sensitive to cold and it "warms up."
- Defective sodium channels do not close properly, leading to continuing influx of sodium molecules into the muscle cells and escape of potassium from these cells. This unwanted depolarization of cell membrane is responsible for myotonia.
- Sodium channelopathy is an autosomal dominant disease and is rarely asymptomatic. Retrospectively, most patients report cold intolerance and muscle cramping and worsening muscle stiffness during exercises.
- Amplitude of CMAP decreases with exercise and exposure to cold.
- Mexiletine is a potent sodium channel blocker that is shown to be effective in non-dystrophic myotonia.

CHAPTER 22

PSEUDONEUROLOGIC SYNDROMES

CASE 22.1: MUSCLE SPASMS AND FACIAL NUMBNESS

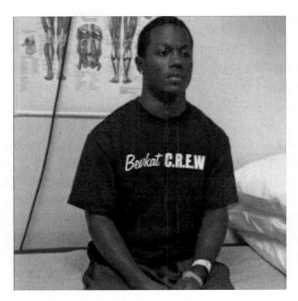

VIDEO 22.1

The patient is an 18-year-old man who is a student athlete at the University of Missouri. His mother's car was hijacked while his mother was visiting him. The mother decided accordingly to move him to Sam Houston University in Houston. Since then he developed muscle spasms that occurred 20 times a day. He also had feet, hand, and facial numbness and poor balance with normal electromyogram (EMG).

The demonstrated signs suggest:

1. Polyminimyoclonus
2. Essential tremor
3. Ataxic neuropathy
4. Functional tremor
5. Stiff person syndrome

DIAGNOSIS

Functional tremor (FT):

The following factors suggest the diagnosis of functional tremor:

1. Acute onset
2. Episodic nature
3. Distractibility
4. It is a mixture of resting, postural, and action tremor.
5. It is irregular.
6. The patient was not responsive during the shaking episode. He was coherent right after with no "post-ictal confusion" to suggest seizure.
7. The tremor resolved spontaneously after he settled into the new college.

- Discussion of pseudoneurologic disorders (PNDs) is beyond the scope of this atlas. The most common PNDs in neuromuscular clinic are functional gait disorder (FGD) and tremor.
- FGD may present with monoplegia, hemiplegia, or paraplegia.
- Hysterical gait can be dramatic, with patients lurching widely in all directions without falling. Examination of the sensory-motor system, cerebellar system, and extrapyramidal system fail to reveal an explanation.
- Normal pressure hydrocephalus (NPH) may be misdiagnosed as FGD when dementia and urinary incontinence are not prominent. The presence of normal strength and sensory system enforces this notion.
  - Gait apraxia of NPH tends to be helped by providing cues such as a stick to step over.

CASE 22.2: SPASMS IN A CIDP PATIENT

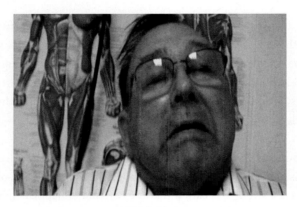

VIDEO 22.2

A 64-year-old man with chronic inflammatory demyelinating polyneuropathy (CIDP) responded to plasmapheresis and azathioprine. He presented with intermittent painless short-lived muscle spasms without alteration of consciousness. No triggers were identified. Brain magnetic resonance imaging (MRI) and electroencephalogram (EEG) were normal.

These episodes are:

1. Related to CIDP exacerbation
2. Seizures
3. Stiff person syndrome
4. Pseudoseizures
5. Neuromuscular

DIAGNOSIS

- Patients with legitimate neuromuscular disorders may develop functional symptoms thoroughout the course of their disease. A neuromuscular specialist therefore may be called to see non-neuromuscular functional disorders in their patients. The first task is to look for any relationship between the new symptoms and their chronic neuromuscular disorder. The second task is to look for an organic explanation for the new symptoms. A good knowledge of psychogenic movement disorders is very helpful to neuromuscular specialists.

- Intermittent posturing and apparent alteration of mental status is a common functional disorder that is hard to differentiate from seizures. The preservation of orientation during these episodes is a strong indication that they are not epileptics. Simple partial seizures by definition are not associated with mental status change, but they are not generalized. Frontal lobe seizures may mimic pseudoseizures (pseudopseudoseizures), and only monitoring with depth electrodes can resolve this confusion. Other features that should suggest pseudoseizures are:
    1. Tip tongue biting
    2. Pelvic thrusting
    3. No postictal confusion
    4. Situational occurrence
    5. Mental coherence during episode
    6. Reactive pupils during episodes
    7. Post-ictal whispering
    8. Closed mouth during the tonic phase
    9. Resisted lid opening
    10. Convulsion lasting more than 2 minutes

- Self-injury and urinary incontinence, contrary to common belief, are not very helpful in differentiating seizures from pseudoseizures, as they occur in both.

CASE 22.3: TREMOR AFTER DIVORCE

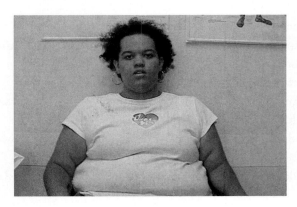

VIDEO 22.3

A 21-year-old woman who was recently divorced, was referred for feet numbness, generalized weakness, and shaking. EMG was normal. She had "give way" weakness and hyperreflexia.

This is a case of:

1. Essential tremor (ET)
2. Parkinson disease (PD)
3. Neuropathy
4. Psychogenic tremor
5. Multiple sclerosis

DIAGNOSIS

- Functional tremor is a common pseudoneurological disorder.
- It usually occurs suddenly and reaches maximum disability fast, unlike organic tremors (ET, PD, cerebellar tremors).
- It ameliorates with distraction and worsens with stress.
- It is constant and not resting, action, or intentional.
- It may affect abdominal muscles.
- Most patients do not have evidence of conversion reaction, but depression seems to be the main associated psychopathology.
- Some patients display other functional symptoms such as gait disorder.

CASE 22.4: QUADRIPLEGIA WITH NORMAL EMG

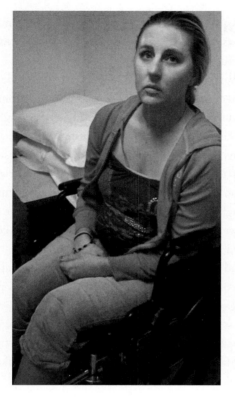

VIDEO 22.4

A 34-year-old woman presented with a 2-year history of subacute quadriplegia and generalized numbness with normal reflexes, creatine kinase (CK) level, cerebrospinal fluid (CSF) examination, brain and spinal cord MRIs, and EMG. Her symptoms were fluctuating and started after she became divorced.

This is a case of:

1. Chronic inflammatory demyelinating polyneuropathy
2. Myopathy
3. Multiple sclerosis
4. Hysterical conversion
5. Myasthenia gravis

DIAGNOSIS

- According to classical Freudian theory, psychological stress may be converted to physical symptoms such as paralysis, blindness, and deafness, or it may dissociate to cognitive symptoms such as mutism and fugue.
- According to Pavlov, severe excitation in the frontal region due to stress leads to reciprocal inhibition of other cortical areas, leading to lack of function.
- "Hysteria" is derived from *hystera* (uterus), as the Greeks thought that the uterus wanders in the body and produces symptoms wherever it settles.
- Charcot rejected this theory; instead, he noted ovarian congestion and tenderness in the victims of "hysteria" and accordingly speculated that the ovaries are the source.
- It is not clear how stress is converted to specific physical symptoms in different people, but it is widely thought that by doing so, it provides a defensive mechanism.
- Clinically, pseudo weakness can be challenging, and it may take the form of mono, hemi, para, or quadriplegia.
- Normal reflexes and sensation and the lack of physiological pattern are clues to the non-organic nature of the deficit, and a normal EMG of weak muscles indicates that the lesion is central (organic or functional).
- "Give way" weakness is highly suggestive of a functional etiology. It is a stepwise loss of resistance of the weak muscles, unlike the smooth loss of resistance in real weakness.
- Both agonist and antagonist muscles are affected equally, unlike organic weakness.
- Unexpected painful stimulation of the affected extremity may lead to purposeful withdrawal.
- Dropping the paralyzed arm on the face leads to "near miss" slap of the face.
- Hoover test: the examiner puts his hand under the heel of the weak side and the other arm on the top of the other leg. Pushing the normal leg against resistance leads to pressure felt by the hand under the heel of the weak leg in cases of pseudoweakness. The examiner then switches hands to verify.
- Adductor sign: Normally, ipsilateral thigh adduction leads to contralateral thigh adduction. The examiner palpates both thigh adductors and asks the patient to adduct the normal side. Contraction of the contralateral (weak) thigh adductors would suggest a functional weakness.
- Some cases of conversion paralysis are chronic, and the benefit of paralysis to draw attention and care unconsciously perpetuates the paralysis.

REFERENCE

Shaibani A, et al. Pseudoneurologic syndromes: recognition and diagnosis. *Am Fam Physician*. 1998;May 15;57(10):2485–2494.

CASE 22.5: "GIVE WAY" WEAKNESS AND LOSS OF BALANCE

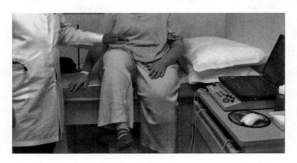

VIDEO 22.5

A 34-year-old woman presented with a 1-month history of tremor, insomnia, generalized fatigue, numbness, and myalgia. She is referred for neuromuscular evaluation of leg weakness. Examination is shown.

The demonstrated proximal weakness is likely due to:

1. Myopathy
2. CIDP
3. Myalgia
4. Psychogenic cause
5. Hip arthritis

DIAGNOSIS

- The term "give way" weakness is used to describe weakness that does not follow a normal smooth yield to resistance; it is mostly functional.
- It can be stepwise, clasp knife, or collapsing weakness (sudden loss of resistance by even touching the weak extremity).
- It takes experience to be able to detect this kind of weakness from the first examination attempt.
- Fortunately, like in this case, there are many clues to the pseudo nature of the weakness, including:
  1. Multiple other symptoms that do not make sense neurologically, like the inability to open mouth and the pseudo right facial weakness.
  2. History of depression or current stress.
  3. La belle indifference: the patient is not much concerned about the symptoms.
- Hyperreflexia is common in this group of patients due to anxiety, and it should not argue against the functional nature of the deficit. Unless it is associated with more objective upper motor neuron (UMN) signs like Babinski sign and spasticity.

CASE 22.6: DYSARTHRIA AFTER A CAR ACCIDENT

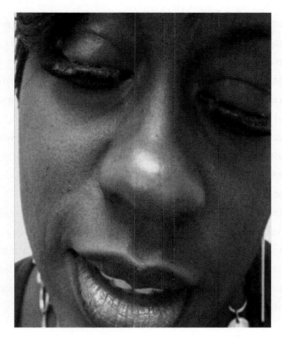

VIDEO 22.6

A 27-year-old woman was referred for neuromuscular evaluation for dysarthria that started 6 weeks earlier after a car accident. There was no dysphagia but she had feet numbness, blurred vision, and generalized weakness. She improved minutes after intramuscular injection of normal saline.

This dysarthria is due to:

1. Amyotrophic lateral sclerosis (ALS)
2. Head injury
3. Psychogenic etiology
4. Cerebellar stroke
5. Myasthenia gravis (MG)

DIAGNOSIS

- Functional speech disorders are common, and some patients are referred to neuromuscular clinics because of suspicion of neuromuscular disorders such as ALS and MG. They include functional mutism, dysphona, and dysarthria.
  - Mutism literally means the inability to speak. Discussing infantile mutism and selective mutism are beyond the scope of this book. In adults, mutism is usually a dissociation hysterical reaction.
  - Dysphonia is a disturbance of phonation and may lead to a whispery voice. Spasmodic dysphonia should not be confused with functional dysphonia. Patients with functional dysphonia may be diagnosed with laryngitis first.
  - Dysarthria may also be psychogenic.
    - The most important features of functional dysarthria are hesitation of pronunciation, especially of sounds in the middle of the words, and being diffuse and involving a combination of lingual, labial, palatal, and laryngeal components.
- Reversal with placebo is typically seen in functional disorders as seen in this case, which responded to normal saline injection. However, the legal and ethical implications of administration of placebo are to be worked out.

CASE 22.7: WEAKNESS AFTER FLU SHOT

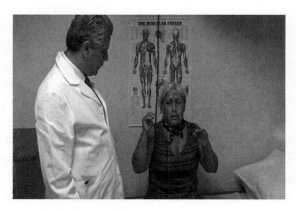

VIDEO 22.7

A 52-year-old woman referred to our neuromuscular clinic due to inability to lift her arms for a year. This started after a flu shot that she believed was a swine flu shot. Deltoid strength was difficult to evaluate due to severe shoulders pain. Her biceps and hip flexors were 5/5 and reflexes were normal. CK level and EMG of the proximal muscles were normal. MRI of the shoulders showed high-grade tear of supraspinatus tendons bilaterally and severe supraspinatus tendinopathy.

The proximal weakness that occurred after the flu shot was due to:

1. Myopathy
2. Psychogenic etiology
3. Shoulder arthritis
4. Fibromyalgia
5. Antigen in the vaccination

DIAGNOSIS

- Clinical manifestations of organic diseases are often complicated by sickness behavior, which occurs as an unconscious psychological reaction to illness. The patient probably had mild arthritis of the shoulders for a while. The pain of the flu shot may have made shoulder abduction painful for a couple of days, which has augmented the effect of arthritis. Sickness behavior is responsible for the rest.
- Very often sickness behavior is punctuated by a patient's understanding of his or her condition. A patient with right-hand numbness due to carpal tunnel syndrome (CTS) may develop numbness in the entire right side because of the connection that the patient makes between hand numbness and stroke.
- This patient improved after physical therapy, NSAIDs, and reassurance. She admitted that she had read a lot of information about the flu shots and their side effects.

CASE 22.8: FACIAL WEAKNESS

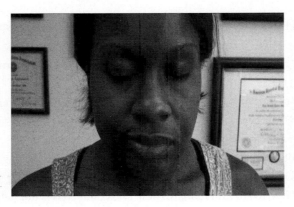

VIDEO 22.8

A 39-year-old woman presented with involuntary movement of the left shoulder and right face, starting after she was fired from work a few weeks earlier. She had facial numbness and pressure like frontal headache. Brain MRI was normal.

The following features suggest psychogenic etiology for the facial spasms, as opposed to hemifacial spasms:

1. Resolution by distraction
2. Frontal headache and facial numbness
3. Worsened by stress
4. Lack of facial weakness
5. Improvement with botulinum toxin injection

DIAGNOSIS

- Patients with HFS are referred to neuromuscular clinics due to a suspicion of facial nerve pathology.
- Jankovic et al. found that 2.4% of cases of HFS seen in their movement disorders clinic had functional HFS.
- The spasms usually starts in the eyelids and are associated with tremor of one or more extremities and with psychological disturbances such as anxiety and depression and other symptoms such as headaches and sensory disturbances.
- Functional HFS usually affects female in their twenties and thirties, while organic HFS affects females in their forties and fifties.
- The use of MRI/MRA to differentiate these two conditions is not helpful because onethird to one-half of organic HFS cases have normal brain MRIs and 15% of brain MRAs control group shows ectasia of the vertebrobasilar system.
- Depression of the ipsilateral eyebrow, elevation of the contralateral eyebrow, and narrowing of the palpebral fissure due to contraction of the upper and lower eyelids are typically seen in functional HFS.
- Most cases resolve within 2 years of the diagnosis.
- Resolution of the spasms by distraction is more typical of functional HFS.
- Both get worse with stress and may get better with botulinum toxin injections and may not be associated with facial weakness.
- Facial numbness and headache suggest an intracranial pathology.

REFERENCE

Tan EK, et al. Psychogenic hemifacial spasm. *The Journal of Neuropsychiatry and Clinical Neurosciences.* 2001;13:380–384.

CHAPTER 23

NUMBNESS

CASE 23.1: INTERCOSTAL BURNING PAIN

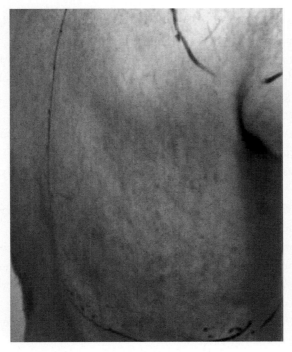

VIDEO 22.1

A 70-year-old man with well-controlled diabetes mellitus (DM) had developed a severe burning sensation and tingling, mostly at rest, along the shown distribution 3 months earlier, which peaked in 5 weeks and plateaued afterward. There was no skin rash, and cervical and thoracic magnetic resonance imaging (MRIs) were normal.

These features suggest:

1. Zoster radiculitis
2. Diabetic thoracoabdominal radiculopathy
3. Myelitis
4. Intercostal neuropathy
5. Non-neuropathic pain

DIAGNOSIS

- This syndrome usually occurs in the context of diabetic lumbosacral radiculoplexus neuropathy (DLSRPN), but it may happen in isolation.
- The pathology is similar to that of DLSRPN and involves microvasculitis rather than metabolic etiology. The disorder occurs in patients with well-controlled DM and no significant end organ damage (retinopathy, nephropathy).
- The pain is neuropathic (burning, occurs mostly at rest) and severe.
- Very often, the diagnosis is not made early and the conditions is misdiagnosed as:
  - Zoster radiculitis:
    - Lack of rash 5 days or more after the onset of pain occurs only in rare cases of the zoster.
    - Diabetic thoraco-abdominal radiculopathy (DTAR) is bilateral in about 30% of cases, which is vanishingly rare in zoster radiculitis.
  - Acute abdomen: appendicitis, cholecystitis, diverticulitis, and so on. Many patients undergo appendectomy or cholecystectomy before they are diagnosed with DTAR.
  - Coronary heart disease: cardiac evaluation is usually done before these patients are referred to a neurologist.
- A key diagnostic feature is skin sensitivity to touch, which is not a feature of acute abdomen or coronary artery disease.
- It is important to rule out compressive and intramedullary lesions by appropriate imaging.
- The condition is self-limiting but it may take 2 years for full recovery.
- Pain management and reassurance are the mainstay of treatment.

CASE 23.2: BURNING PAIN IN A DIABETIC

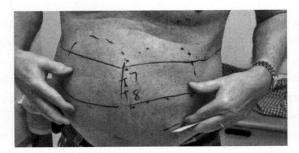

VIDEO 23.2

A 56-year-old man with controlled diabetes mellitus (DM) presented with a 6-month history of severe burning pain that progressively spread in the shown distribution. He used a special elastic T-shirt and bathed with warm water several times a night to reduce pain. His ankle reflexes and feet sensation were normal and entire spinal cord MRI was normal.

The pathology of this syndrome is likely due to:

1. Metabolic axonal injury
2. Microvasculitis
3. Compressive neuropathy
4. Drug-induced intercostal neuropathy
5. Secondary viral infection

DIAGNOSIS

- Pathologically, diabetic neuropathies are classified into those that are caused by:
  - Metabolic and chronic ischemic changes such as diabetic polyneuropathy, and those that are caused by
  - Acute or subacute microvasculitis. This category is characterized by acute or subacute pain and focal or multifocal involvement. The following discussion is about the second category.
- The pain is severe but self-limiting. EMG usually shows evidence of multifocal axonal neuropathy.
- These patients usually have good diabetes control and no evidence of end organ damage.
- Recovery process may take months to years.
- Examples of this group of diabetic neuropathies include:
  - Diabetic third cranial nerve palsy
  - Diabetic thoracoabdominal radiculopathy
  - Diabetic lumbosacral radiculoplexus neuropathy
- Detailed pathological studies demonstrated multifocal fiber loss, perineurial thickening, neovascularization, perivascular inflammation, and invasion of small blood vessels wall with mononuclear inflammatory cells consistent with microvasculitis. The cause of this inflammatory pathology is not clear.

REFERENCE

Dyck PJ, Norell JE, Dyck PJ. Microvasculitis and ischemia in diabetic lumbosacral radiculoplexus neuropathy. *Neurology.* 1999;53:2113–2121.

CASE 23.3: PATCHY SENSORY LOSS

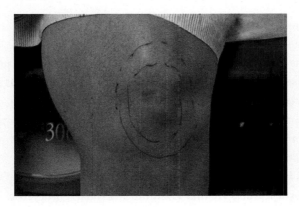

VIDEO 23.3

A 51-year-old woman presented with sequential patchy sensory loss and no evidence of polyneuropathy.

These symptoms are typical of:

1. Psychogenic etiology
2. Diabetic radiculopathy
3. Zoster radiculitis
4. Migrant sensory neuritis of Wartenberg
5. None of the above

DIAGNOSIS

Migrant sensory neuritis of Wartenberg:

- This syndrome is characterized by recurrent episodes of burning pain and subsequent patchy loss of sensation in the distribution of one cutaneous nerve at a time.
- It mostly affects the skin of the extremities, chest, and face.
- These sensory changes are usually induced by movement of a limb or pressure on the skin, by kneeling for example, leading to stretching of a cutaneous nerve.
- It usually affects people in their fourth or fifth decade.
- It is described as a pure sensory mononeuritis multiplex.
- Electrodiagnostic features are that of multifocal axonal sensory loss.
- Biopsy of affected nerves show findings suggestive of an autoimmune vascular process including:
  - Perineurial scarring
  - Chronic inflammation
  - Axonal loss and regeneration
  - Differential fascicular involvement
  - Endoneurial edema
  - Immunoglobulin deposition
- The effect of immunomodulation on the course of the disease is ill defined, especially as the disorder is purely sensory and does not cause functional impairment other than pain.
- No association is reported between this condition and diabetes mellitus or autoimmune disorders.

CASE 23.4: FEET NUMBNESS AND NORMAL ANKLE REFLEXES

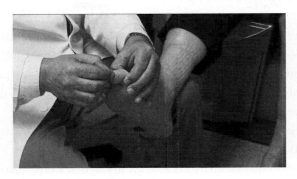

VIDEO 23.4

A 74-year-old healthy man presented with poor balance since age 40 years. Examination is shown. Brain and cervical MRIs are non-contributory.

The most appropriate next diagnostic step is:

1. Thoracic magnetic resonance imaging (MRI)
2. Nerve conduction study/electromyogram (NCS/EMG)
3. Cerebrospinal fluid (CSF) examination
4. Skin biopsy
5. Nerve biopsy

DIAGNOSIS

Feet numbness and normal ankle reflexes:

- An important clinical scenario commonly seen in neuromuscular clinics is patients with chronic progressive sensory ataxia with preserved or brisk ankle reflexes.
- Sensory symptoms in the feet are suspected of being neuropathic when ankle reflexes are decreased or absent. In that case, an NCS is indicated to determine the type and severity of neuropathy.
- However, if the ankle reflexes are brisk or even normal, the following possibilities are to be considered:
  - If feet pain and skin sensitivity to touch are the main features, small fiber neuropathy is an important consideration, and a skin biopsy is indicated.
  - If vibratory and proprioceptive deficits are the main findings, a central lesion is suspected. Cervical myelopathy, compressive or not, is the most common cause, but thoracic myelopathy and intracranial lesions are to be considered if cervical MRI is negative.
    - Myeloneuropathy is also possible; therefore, the presence of neuropathy, even if confirmed by NCS, should not preclude investigating the spinal cord in cases where ankle reflexes are brisk or normal in the face of severe feet numbness.
    - Cervical spondylotic myelopathy with diabetic or non-diabetic neuropathy is a common scenario where feet numbness is associated with brisk ankle jerks.
  - Feet numbness with persevered ankle reflexes should always trigger the need to test for Babinski sign, which if positive would support the presence of a central component.
- This patient was found to have moderate cord compression due to a large arachnoid cyst extending from T3 to T6.

CASE 23.5: FEET PAIN AND ORTHOSTASIS

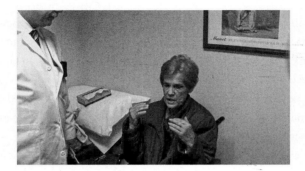

VIDEO 23.5

A 60-year-old woman with no significant past medical history had developed asymmetric progressive pain and numbness of the feet. A month later, she had similar symptoms in the arms and postural hypotension. EMG revealed axonal sensorimotor neuropathy. Autonomic reflexes testing revealed moderate dysautonomia. CSF protein was normal. Sed rate was 43 mm/hr. Serum creatinine was 2.3 mg/dl. IFPE revealed an IgM kappa spike. Left sural nerve biopsy is shown (Figures 23.5.1 and 23.5.2).

Family history is remarkable for neuropathy and DM affecting her father.

The likely diagnosis is:

1. Familial amyloidosis
2. Vasculitis
3. AL amyloidosis
4. Toxic neuropathy
5. Familial autonomic and sensory neuropathy

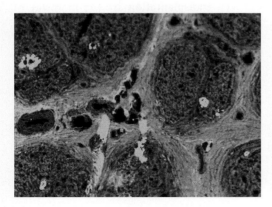

FIGURE 23.5.1 Congo red stain of left sural nerve biopsy viewed under fluorescent light.

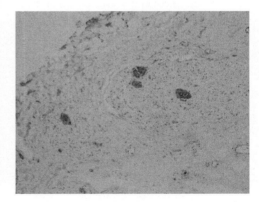

FIGURE 23.5.2 Positive reaction to Kappa chain antibodies.

DIAGNOSIS

- Progressive painful asymmetric or multifocal neuropathy suggests vasculitis or amyloidosis. Dysautonomia is more typical for the later. Renal impairment is common in both conditions.
- Family history suggests familial amyloid neuropathy but monoclonal gammopathy is favorable of AL amyloidosis. Sural nerve biopsy confirmed amyloidosis. The tissue was reacted for different paraproteins and reaction was positive for IgM Kappa short chain, the same protein found in the serum. Transthyretin mutations were negative.
- AL amyloidosis:
  - Amyloid is a misfolded protein in a beta pleated sheet configuration. It is insoluble and is deposited in the extracellular tissue, mostly nerves (axonal neuropathy), kidneys, heart, tongue, carpal tunnel, and small fiber and autonomic fibers.
- A clinical triad of progressive painful neuropathy, bilateral CTS, and dysautonomia is typical for amyloidosis.
- Monoclonal proteins are precursors of amyloid; therefore, their presence, along with progressive painful neuropathy or dysautonomic symptoms, should raise the possibility of AL amyloidosis, especially if there is renal or cardiac involvement.
- AL amyloidosis consists of kappa or lambda misfolded protein.
- Multiple myeloma may present 1–7 years after diagnosis of AL amyloidosis.
- Clinical syndrome of AL amyloidosis:
  - Painful distal symmetric sensory neuropathy
  - Carpal tunnel syndrome (CTS)
  - Dysautonomia: orthostatic hypotension, hyporeactive pupils, anhidrosis, urinary incontinence, impotence.
  - Myopathy
  - Cardiac and renal impairment.
  - It may present as mononeuritis multiplex (usually associated with lymphoma): look for lymphadenopathy.
  - It is a progressive disease and survival is 1–10 years.
  - Renal and cardiac involvement is a bad sign.
  - Chemotherapy and peripheral blood stem cell transplantation are the mainstay of therapy.

CHAPTER 24

DEFORMITIES

CASE 24.1: MYALGIA, WEAKNESS, AND HARD BREASTS

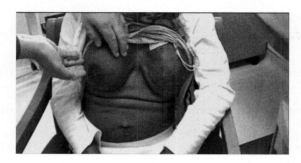

VIDEO 24.1

A 55 year-old woman with uremia treated with hemodialysis, who had received a gadolinium-enhanced brain magnetic resonance imaging (MRI) for neurological symptoms, developed progressive painful inability to raise legs and arms, which was confirmed in the examination. She also had severe hardening of the breasts and thigh tissue. Creatine kinase (CK) level and electromyography (EMG) were normal and non-gadolinium MRI of the thighs revealed sclerosis of the subcutaneous tissue with sparing of the muscles.

The following fact(s) is (are) accurate about nephrogenic systemic sclerosis (NSS):

1. It occurs only in uremic patients who receive gadolinium.
2. It occurs only in dialysis patients.
3. It responds well to cyclophosphamide.
4. It causes fibrosis of internal organs.
5. It does not cause contractures.

DIAGNOSIS

- Nephrogenic systemic sclerosis is a rare condition characterized by fibrosis of skin, joints, and internal organs.
- It is associated with exposure to gadolinium, which is used as a paramagnetic contrast in MRIs.
- Different brands of gadolinium may have different potentials in producing this disorder.
- It is more common in patients with renal failure who are on hemodialysis or peritoneal dialysis.
- Gadolinium is contraindicated when glomerular filtration rate (GFR) is less than 50 ml/min due to progressively increased risk of NSS.
- No other risk factors are identified, and genetic predisposition is suggested.
- Patients present with severe contractures and joint pain.
- Fibrosis may extend to liver, lungs, and heart.
- Pathologically, the fibrotic areas show thickened collagen and proliferation of fibroblasts.
- Skin thickening may resemble scleroderma and systemic sclerosis.
- Neuromuscular involvement is difficult to evaluate due to severe joint and skin fibrosis, but fibrosis of the underlying muscles and myopathic changes are demonstrated by EMG and muscle biopsy in a few patients.
- These patients are referred to neuromuscular clinics due to proximal weakness and suspicion of myopathy.
- No treatment is found to be effective in ameliorating the disease process.

CASE 24.2: CERVICAL DEFORMITY

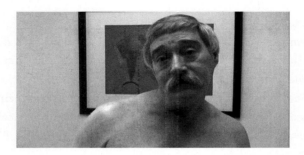

VIDEO 24.2

A 55-year-old man presented with cervical dystonia since childhood, resulting in mechanical cervical deformity confirmed by cervical spine MRI. The patient was referred to the neuromuscular clinic for numbness and spasticity of the legs, which turned out due to myelopathy caused by the mentioned deformity.

Cervical spine mechanical restriction can result from:

1. Long-standing cervical dystonia
2. Periodic familial paralysis
3. Congenital torticollis
4. Head tremor
5. Polymyalgia rheumatica

DIAGNOSIS

- Musculoskeletal deformities (MSDs) are:
  - Important markers for hereditary and congenital neuromuscular diseases.
  - They can also result from dystonia, contractures, and chronic immobility.
- Musculoskeletal deformities (MSDs):
  - Can cause neurological dysfunction themselves, regardless of their origin; the patient in this case developed myelopathy due to dystonia-induced cervical spine deformity.
- The most relevant MSDs in neuromuscular disorders are kyphosis, Pes Cavus, hammer-toes, and high arched palate.
- Pes Cavus is characterized by high feet arches that do not flatten with weight bearing, contrary to the acquired high feet arches that flatten upon weight bearing.
  - 10% of the general population has Pes Cavus.
  - Pes Cavus may represent the earliest manifestations of neuromuscular disorders.
  - Common neuromuscular disorders (NMD) associated with Pes Cavus are hereditary motor and sensory neuropathy (HSMN), spinocerebellar ataxia (SCA), hereditary neuropathy with liability to pressure palsies (HNPP), and congenital myopathies.
  - Pes Cavus occurs due to imbalance between weak intrinsic feet muscles (lumbricals and interossi) and overactive peroneus and tibialis posterior.
  - Family history of Pes Cavus is important to explore because it could be a marker for a hereditary neuromuscular disorder.
- A neuromuscular specialist should make a point to look for MSDs, especially Pes Cavus, and to ask about family history of these deformities, especially in patients with chronic "idiopathic" neuropathies and myopathies.

CASE 24.3: MULTIPLE MASSES AND PROXIMAL WEAKNESS

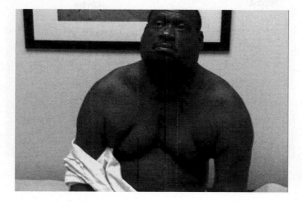

VIDEO 24.3

A 65-year-old man presented with several years history of chronic progressive proximal weakness, loss of balance, feet numbness and myalgia. Two benign masses were removed from his upper back few years earlier. CK level was 356 U/L and EMG showed evidence of myopathy and axonal neuropathy. Muscle biopsy and pedigree are shown (Figures 24.3.1 and 24.3.2).

The most likely unifying diagnosis is:

1. Lymphoma
2. Neurofibromatosis
3. Mitochondrial disease
4. Metastatic cancer
5. None of the above

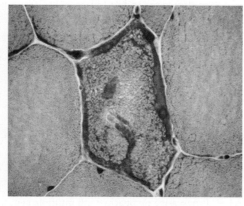

FIGURE 24.3.1 Left biceps muscle biopsy (400x).

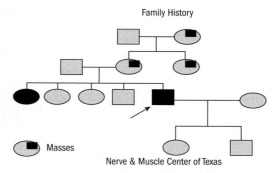

FIGURE 24.3.2 Pedigree of the patient.

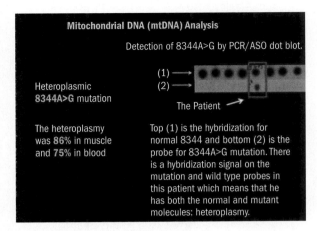

FIGURE 24.3.3 DNA analysis of the patient.

DIAGNOSIS

- These patients are referred to neuromuscular clinics due to proximal weakness and feet numbness.
- The video shows several masses in the clavicular area and chest wall.
- Muscle biopsy showed ragged red fibers, suggestive of mitochondrial dysfunction.
- Myopathy, neuropathy, multiple soft masses, and ragged red fibers suggest Madelung disease.
- Genetics is complicated. Most cases are due to mitochondrial mutations, but some are autosomal dominant while others are sporadic.
- Middle-aged men with a history of alcoholism are typically affected.
- Multiple fatty swelling in the proximal arms and legs, back of neck, side of neck, around shoulders, and supraclavicular areas is usually noted.
- Distal symmetric axonal sensorimotor neuropathy is common.
- EMG usually shows non-irritative proximal myopathy and distal axonal neuropathy.
- Autonomic reflexes are abnormal with evidence of dysautonomia.
- Mild CK elevation is usually seen, and muscle biopsy shows ragged red fibers.
- Surgical removal of lipomas to relieve compression or for cosmetic reason can be attempted, but recurrence is common.
- The mitochondrial variant is associated with A8344G mutation in mitochondrial tRNA^{Lys} (Figure 24.3.3).
- Some families also have myoclonic epilepsy with ragged red fibers (MERRF) syndrome.

REFERENCE

Brunetti-Pierri N, Shaibani A, Zhang S, Wong LJ, Shinawi M. Progressive myopathy with multiple symmetric lipomatosis. *Arch Neurol.* 2009 Dec;66(12):1576–1577.

CHAPTER 25

FATIGABILITY

CASE 25.1: FATIGABILITY OF SPEECH

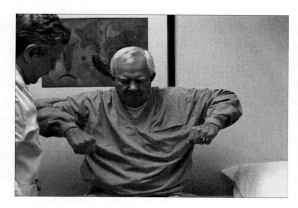

VIDEO 25.1

A 62-year-old man presented with a 6-month history of slurring of speech and undue fatigability of the arm and leg muscles.

Fatigability in myasthenia gravis (MG) affects:

1. Biceps more than triceps
2. Neck extensors more than neck flexors
3. Superior oblique more than superior recti
4. Wrist extensors more than wrists flexors
5. 2 and 4

DIAGNOSIS

- Clinical examination for fatigability is often omitted from the neurological examination. Right deltoid muscle is fatigable in this patient.
- Patients with weakness and or fatigue, especially if they have ocular and or bulbar symptoms, should always be asked about undue fatigability and worsening of symptoms in the evenings and improvement with rest.
- Occurrence of diplopia with reading and watching TV and toward the end of the day is an important diagnostic finding in myasthenia gravis (MG).
- It is important to know that fatigue is a natural phenomenon and is increased with age.
- Most neurological motor disorders cause undue fatigability, such as myopathies and amyotrophic lateral sclerosis (ALS).
- The most common causes of fatigue in medicine are non-neuromuscular and include disorders such as:
  - Anemia
  - Hypothyroidism
  - Obstructive sleep apnea
  - Depression
- MG is an important but a rare cause of undue fatigability.
- Problematic cases occur when generalized fatigability is associated with negative myasthenia serology and with no ocular and or bulbar symptoms. Chronic fatigue syndrome becomes a consideration after medical and psychological causes are ruled out.
  - In chronic fatigue syndrome (CFS), fatigue is almost constant and it does not fluctuate clearly.
- In MG, fatigue affects extensors more than flexors and elevators more than depressors of the eyes.
  - Neck extensors are differentially affected and are much more fatigable than neck flexors, unlike myopathies.
  - Triceps are more affected than biceps, especially in African Americans.
  - Wrist extensors and ankle dorsiflexors can be so severely affected that wrist drop and foot drop may result.
- Fatigue and weakness are used interchangeably by patients. It is important to ask about them separately. Weakness is a motor inability that is present since the start of the movement and it may or may not fatigue. Fatigability on the other hand is weakness that happens only with use and recovers to baseline or close to baseline with rest.
- In severe cases, fatigue may become a fixed weakness; on the other hand, mild weakness may fatigue with use, creating overlap between weakness and fatigue.

CASE 25.2: FATIGABLE NECK MUSCLES

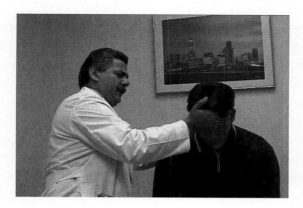

VIDEO 25.2

A 30-year-old man presented with fatigable ptosis and diplopia. Examination is shown. Fatigability of muscles in myasthenia gravis (MG) occurs due to:

1. Progressive loss of contractile elements
2. Reduction of the safety factor
3. Decreased quantal acetylcholine release with successive stimuli at intervals greater than 500 seconds
4. Blocking of increasing numbers of muscle fibers
5. Does not affect the external anal sphincter

DIAGNOSIS

- The video shows right ptosis and fatigability of the neck flexion with restoration after rest.
- Fatigue is a complex phenomenon that is regulated by central and peripheral factors. As far as the neuromuscular junction (NMJ) is concerned, the clinically and neurophysiologically detected fatigue pattern can be understood on the basis of normal physiology:
  - A nerve action potential leads to fusion of acetylcholine (ACh) vesicles to presynaptic membrane (docking), followed by release of neurotransmitter (ACh) from vesicles into the synaptic cleft and attachment of ACh to post-synaptic ACh receptors (AChR). This leads to stimulation of the postsynaptic membrane, resulting in a generation of end plate potential (EPP) that usually exceeds 50 mV. This EPP is three to four times more than what is needed by a muscle fiber (10–15 mV) to depolarize from its resting membrane potential (safety margin).
  - Repetitive stimulation at frequency of 5 Hz **normally** depletes ACh-containing vesicles.
  - After 4 stimulations, the ACh release is resuscitated by newly arriving ACh from the presynaptic terminal.
  - After a minute, the ACh release is reduced due to decreased availability.
- Reduction of postsynaptic acetylcholine receptors AChR due to antibody reaction leads to reduced amplitude of the end plate potential (EPP) safety margin to a level that is barely enough to produce an action potential in the beginning of the exercise but cannot maintain that when the normal decline in the release occurs, leading to block of muscle fibers and consequently fatigue.
- Quantal release is not affected in MG but in presynaptic neuromuscular disorders.
- External anal sphincter consists of skeletal muscles and therefore it is affected by fatigue in MG. Patients, especially female, with pelvic floor weakness may rely on external anal sphincter to prevent "leaks."
- The right answer is 2, 4

CASE 25.3: MYASTHENIA AND ELEVATED CK LEVEL

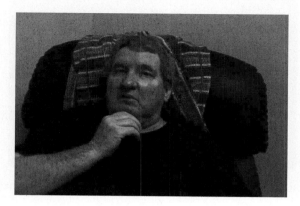

VIDEO 25.3

A 60-year-old man presented with severe chewing difficulty. There was no ptosis or diplopia. He developed subacute proximal weakness. Examination is shown. Acetylcholine receptors antibody (AChR Ab) titer was 25 nml/l and creatine kinase (CK) was 5,000 U/L. Electromyography (EMG) revealed 40% short duration units in the proximal leg and arm muscles and many fibrillations and positive sharp waves. Computed tomography (CT) of the chest showed a mediastinal mass.

A muscle biopsy will likely show:

1. Lymphorrhagia
2. Granulomatous myositis
3. Caseating granulomata
4. Perimysial inflammation
5. Perifascicular atrophy

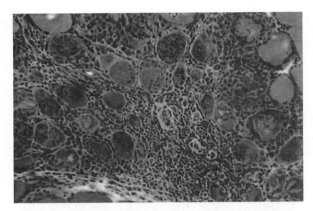

FIGURE 25.3.1 H&E stain (400x): Endomysial non-caseating granuloma with many multinucleated giant cells.

DIAGNOSIS

- Examination showed fatigability of the muscles of mastication and dysarthria.
- Increased CK level, irritative myopathy, and mediastinal mass suggest giant cells myositis (GCM).
- GCM is a rare form of polymyositis that is usually associated with thymoma and carditis.
- Myositis can occur before or after the diagnosis of myasthenia gravis (MG) and thymoma.
- GCM has less favorable prognosis than polymyositis, due to frequent cardiac involvement.
- The formation of granuloma suggests cell-mediated immunity.
- The frequent occurrence of MG suggests humeral immunity.
- The initial presentation of subacute fatigable dysarthria and dysphagia was consistent with MG, but the following factors raised the possibility of polymyositis (PM) and promoted a muscle biopsy and CT scan of the chest:
  1. HyperCKemia: mild CK elevation is not inconsistent with MG. More than five times normal CK level is atypical.
  2. More severe proximal weakness than expected for MG
  3. More irritaitve myopathic units proximally than expected for MG
- This patient had a thymectomy 15 years ago and he continues to enjoy a normal life, but relapsed every time azathioprine or prednisone was discontinued. Thymoma did not recur.

CASE 25.4: INABILITY TO CHEW A STEAK

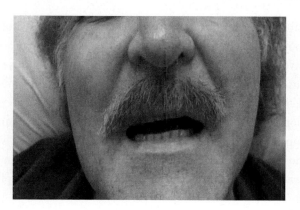

VIDEO 25.4

A 54-year-old man presented with an inability to chew without supporting his chin with his hand. There was no pain.

The most likely diagnosis is:

1. Temporal arteritis
2. Temporomandibular joint (TMJ) dysfunction
3. Myasthenia gravis (MG)
4. Psychogenic
5. Mandibular dystonia

DIAGNOSIS

- Painless fatigability of the muscles of mastication is characteristic of myasthenia gravis. The patient could not close his mouth completely and he had left ptosis.
- Sometimes, involvement of the jaw muscles is severe enough to cause jaw ptosis.
- Patients may use their hands to support their jaws during mastication and even talking.
- They cannot keep their mouths shut and their eyes open.
- Jaw claudication, on the other hand, is the inability to chew due to pain, and it is typically caused by temporal arteritis, which can cause ophthalmoplegia as well, adding another layer of diagnostic confusion. Vasculitic changes of the arterial supply of the mastication muscles and extraocular muscles (EOM) is the pathological explanation of pain and opthalmoplegia.
- Pyridostigmine, an hour before meals, may improve chewing function.
- Fatigability of the chewing muscles usually improves smoothly, along with the other features of myasthenia, with treatment.

CASE 25.5: CASE 25.4 AFTER TREATMENT WITH PLASMA EXCHANGE (PLEX)

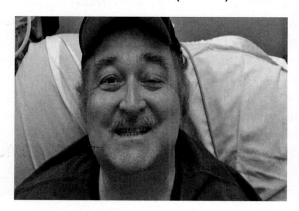

VIDEO 25.5

After five sessions of plasmapheresis (PLEX), the patient could close his mouth completely and chew solid food without using his hands.

Plasmapheresis in myasthenia gravis:

1. Is equally effective to intravenous immunoglobulin (IVIG)
2. Is superior to intravenous immunoglobulin (IVIG) in the long run
3. Is preferred over IVIG in patients with congestive heart failure (CCF)
4. Is less effective than IVIG
5. Is preferred over IVIG in HIV patients

DIAGNOSIS

- Plasmapheresis is shown to be as effective as intravenous immunoglobulin (IVIG) in the treatment of myasthenia gravis (MG). A close look at the temporal profile of improvement indicates that plasmapheresis worked faster.
- Due to perceived complications and technical difficulty in obtaining venous access, most experts use plasma exchange (PLEX) for the following indications:
  1. Myasthenic crisis
  2. To prepare for major surgery
  3. Long-term treatment in refractory cases
  4. When IVIG is associated with high risk such as in patients with congestive cardiac failure
- Clinical improvement may appear as soon as the third day of treatment.
- Complications of plasma exchange (PLEX) occur in 10% of sessions, and they are usually mild and treatable.
- Most complications are related to the vascular access and include obstruction, infection, and thrombosis.
- Procedure-related complications include hypotension, anemia, hypokalemia, and arrhythmias.
- Patients who need a long-term treatment may benefit from arteriovenous fistula (AVF).

REFERENCE

Ebadi H, et al. Safety of plasma exchange therapy in patients with myasthenia gravis. *Muscle and Nerve.* 2013;47:510–514.

CASE 25.6: FATIGABILITY OF TRICEPS MUSCLE

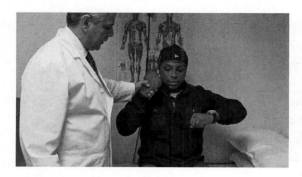

VIDEO 25.6

A 35-year-old man with seropositive generalized myasthenia gravis (MG) had responded well to steroids and azathioprine. However, he did not regain the ability to do bench presses, even 3 years later, and he had to give up his favorite sport.

Weakness of triceps muscles in this case is:

1. Due to MG
2. Argues against MG
3. Due to myopathy
4. Due to C7 radiculopathy
5. Persistence is against the diagnosis of MG

DIAGNOSIS

- Weakness of triceps is common in MG but is only reported when it is severe or interferes with activity.
- African American myasthenics may have more incidence of triceps weakness than other races.
- It is a good habit for neuromuscular specialists to include triceps in their examination for weakness and fatigability in patients with myasthenia gravis.
- Residual weakness of triceps is not uncommon.

CLINICAL SIGNS

CASE 26.1: EYE MOVEMENT

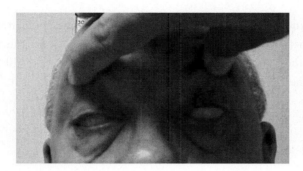

VIDEO 26.1

A 65-year-old man presented with bilateral facial weakness.
The demonstrated upward eye movement is called:

1. Doll's eye movement
2. Bell phenomenon
3. Roving eye movement
4. Oculogyric crisis
5. Leuco-ophthalmia

DIAGNOSIS

- Bell phenomenon is an upward movement of the eye globes with attempted forceful eye closure or when the cornea is touched. It is a normal defensive function and occurs in about 75% of the population. The rolling of the eyeballs is more readily visible when there is facial weakness (e.g., Guillain-Barré syndrome, Bell palsy, etc.).

CASE 26.2: SWEATING DURING PREACHING

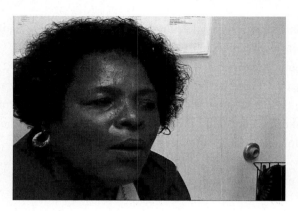

VIDEO 26.2

A 54-year-old preacher had to quit preaching due to embarrassing drenching facial sweating during preaching. She had no other features of dysautonomia and her examination was normal.

The following treatments are used for primary facial hyperhidrosis:

1. Anticholinergic medications
2. Sympathectomy
3. Botulinum toxin injection
4. Steroids
5. 1, 2, and 3

DIAGNOSIS

- Drenching facial sweating provoked by stress is not uncommon, leading to social embarrassment and impairment of ability to work.
- Obesity and female sex are risk factors.
- Focal increase of sweating in the axilla and palms can be disturbing as well.
- To determine the actual dimension of the condition and the area of hyperhidrosis, the patient was asked to recreate the precipitating condition. This also helped define the area needed to be injected with botulinum.
- This case provides a lesson on the importance of reproducing physical signs in the office whenever the physical signs are scarce compared to the symptoms.

CASE 26.3: FACILITATED REFLEXES

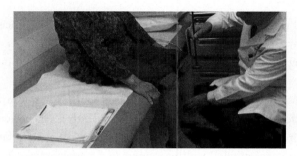

VIDEO 26.3

A 65-year-old woman presented with a 7-month history of fatigue and difficulty arising out of a chair. She lost 20 pounds and developed brownish pigmentation of the skin. Her examination revealed proximal weakness and the mentioned finding.

The most likely diagnosis is:

1. Myopathy
2. Lambert-Eaton myasthenic syndrome (LEMS)
3. Myasthenia gravis (MG)
4. Proximal motor neuropathy
5. Anxiety

DIAGNOSIS

- Facilitation of reflexes after exercising the related muscles (quadriceps in this case) is a feature of presynaptic neuromuscular transmission (NMT) disorder. It is similar to facilitation of strength with repeated testing and facilitation of the compound action potential with exercise.
- Areflexia is an important diagnostic criterion of Lambert-Eaton myasthenic syndrome (LEMS) beside proximal weakness and fatigue and only 6% of patients do not display it.
- Transient improvement of strength after exercise is due to accumulation of calcium ions in the presynaptic terminals, resulting in increased acetylcholine (Ach) release.
- This sign is only seen in a third of patients with Lambert-Eaton myasthenic syndrome (LEMS); therefore, its absence should not be held against the diagnosis.
- Since LEMS patients usually present with proximal weakness similar to myopathy, the lack of deep tendon reflexes (DTRs) and facilitation of reflexes with exercises should raise the possibility of LEMS in these patients.

CASE 26.4: RESTLESS LEGS

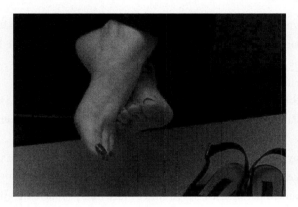

VIDEO 26.4

A 60-year-old woman presented with restlessness and insomnia due to an irresistible desire to move her feet that occurred for decades and responded intermittently to pramipexole. She had no evidence of neuropathy or lumbosacral (LS) radiculopathy. Her hemoglobin was 12 gm/dl. She had two sisters with the same problem.

This is a case of:

1. Parkinson disease (PD)
2. Neuropathy
3. Muscle cramps
4. Restless leg syndrome (RLS)
5. Akathisia

DIAGNOSIS

- Restless leg syndrome (RLS) is a common disorder and affects 5%–10% of population.
- It is characterized by the urgent and irresistible desire to move the legs and sometimes arms.
- Patients describe such a desire as tingling or cramping.
- It should be differentiated from other "urge to move" disorders like akathisia.
- Differential diagnosis includes polyneuropathy and legs cramps that can lead to secondary RLS.
- Iron deficiency anemia is commonly associated with RLS. Low brain iron is shown to interfere with dopaminergic pathway.
- Family members of patients are seven times more likely to have the disorder than the rest of the population.
- 60% of cases are familial. It is inherited as an autosomal dominant disorder with variable penetrance. At least three genetic loci are identified. A genetic control of the dopaminergic system is well established.
- Worsening of leg movement at rest and nighttime and improvement with movement is an important diagnostic feature.
- 80% of cases are associated with periodic limb movement.
- Dopamine agonists are only indicated in severe cases and they may cause paradoxical worsening.

CASE 26.5: HYPERREFLEXIA

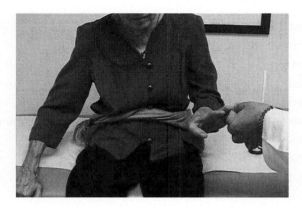

VIDEO 26.5

A 77-year-old woman presented with chronic cervical pain, numbness of the hands, stiffness of the legs, and urinary frequency. She had atrophy and weakness of the hand muscles.

The demonstrated sign is named after:

1. Babinski
2. Hoffmann
3. Lhermitte
4. Uhthoff
5. Chaddock

DIAGNOSIS

- Tapping the nail or flicking the terminal phalanx of the ipsilateral ring finger produces sudden and transient flexion of the thumb and index finger.
- Hoffmann sign can be normal, especially in hyperreflexic individuals.
- It is more significant if unilateral and is consistent with upper motor neuron injury such as cervical myelopathy and amyotrophic lateral sclerosis (ALS).
- It is called "Babinski sign of the arm," but it is a deep tendon reflex (monosynaptic), unlike Babinski sign, which is a polysynaptic reflex.
- Babinski sign is always abnormal except in infants.

CASE 26.6: POOR ARMS ABDUCTION

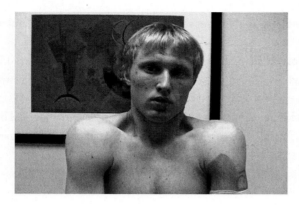

VIDEO 26.6

A 24-year-old man presented with an inability to raise his arms despite good deltoid strength since age 15 years.

There are enough clinical findings to strongly suggest:

1. Myotonic dystrophy
2. Facioscapulohumeral muscular dystrophy (FSHD)
3. Duchenne muscular dystrophy
4. Bilateral phrenic palsy supraspinatous weakness
5. Severe shoulder arthritis

DIAGNOSIS

- There are several physical findings that suggest facioscapulohumeral muscular dystrophy (FSHD).
- Atrophy of pectoralis is an early sign.
- Normally, clavicles are pulled down by the pectoralis muscles (red arrow, Figure 26.6.1) and hence a weak pectoralis leads to "horizontal clavicles."
- The axillary folds are formed by the pectoralis and they are diagonal lines moving toward the humerus (black arrow Figure 26.6.1). When pectoralis is wasted, these folds are "reversed."
- Inability to raise arms despite preservation of supraspinatus and deltoids is due to scapular instability.
- The presence of pumps and depressions resulting from protruded bones and preserved muscles (deltoid, brachioradialis) alternating with small muscles (biceps and pectoralis) is called "poly-hill sign."
- The patient also has mild facial weakness and scapular winging.
- Symptoms of FSHD can be subtle and can escape diagnosis for years.

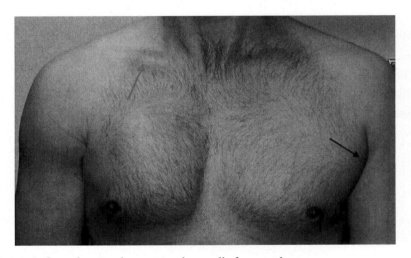

FIGURE 26.6.1 A photo showing the anterior chest wall of a normal person.

CASE 26.7: TENSILON TEST

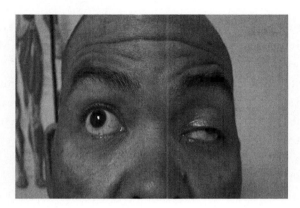

VIDEO 26.7

A 60-year-old man presented with a 6-month history of diplopia. The second half of the recording was taken right after IV injection of 10 mg of edrophonium and shows improvement of the ptosis and left medial rectus strength.

Improvement of ptosis with edrophonium is:

1. Specific for myasthenia gravis (MG)
2. Is 90% sensitive for MG
3. Occurs after 10 minutes of administration
4. Lasts 2 hours
5. None of the above

DIAGNOSIS

- Edrophonium chloride (Tensilon) inhibits acetylcholine esterase. It is short acting.
- Tensilon test is used to confirm the diagnosis of myasthenia gravis (MG). It is 90% sensitive but is only 60% specific.
- False positive test can be seen in Lambert-Eaton myasthenic syndrome (LEMS), amyotrophic lateral sclerosis (ALS), and neuropathies, and is due to increased neuromuscular junction irritability in these conditions.
- The procedure is performed as following:
  - A vein is cannulated and 2 mg of edrophonium chloride (EC) is injected to test for allergy. Within 2 minutes, 8 mg of the same is pushed.
  - A response is expected in 2–5 minutes. Increased salivation and lacrimation are signs of action.
  - The test is not as valuable if there are no clear outcome measures such as a significant ptosis or tropia.
  - Some experts advocate for a control arm of the test to rule out a placebo effect.
  - The pulse rate (PR) and the blood pressure (BP) should be monitored since bradycardia and hypotension can occur. Atropine should be available on standby for emergencies.
  - The duration of action is only few minutes.
- The use of this test has become limited after the introduction of serological and neurophysiological tests for myasthenia gravis (MG), but it still has a place in ocular myasthenia gravis (OMG), where these tests are not very sensitive.
- In this case, the movement of the left medial rectus (MR) and left ptosis improved with Tensilon.

CASE 26.8: SENSORY TRICKS

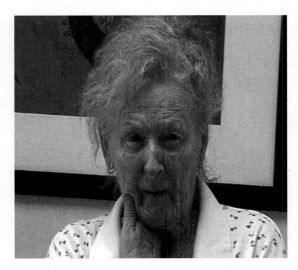

VIDEO 26.8

A 65-year-old woman presented with oromandibular dystonia.

The reason the patient is touching her face and lips with the finger is:

1. A random habit
2. To provide tactile stimulation to alleviate dystonia
3. To minimize pain
4. To taste and smell her finger
5. To express shyness

DIAGNOSIS

- Many movement disorders are characterized by amelioration by sensory tricks.
- Cervical dystonia and blepharospasm are more affected by these tricks than hemifacial spasm and writer's cramps.
- Among the sensory tricks, tactile stimulation is the most common trick. The mechanism is not clear. Somehow, sensory input from the affected area modulates motor output to the involved muscles.

REFERENCE

Loyola DP, Camargos S, Maia D, Cardoso F. Sensory tricks in focal dystonia and hemifacial spasm. *Eur J Neurol.* 2013 Apr;20(4):704–707. doi:10.1111/ene.12054. Epub 2012 Dec 7.

CASE 26.9: OPTIC NEURITIS AND MYELOPATHY

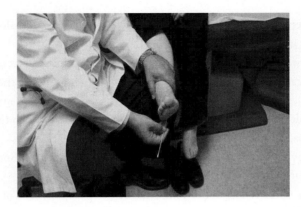

VIDEO 26.9

A 40-year-old woman presented with recurrent transverse myelitis and optic neuritis. The demonstrated signs include all the following except:

1. Babinski
2. Chaddock
3. Oppenheim
4. Hoffman
5. Uhthoff

DIAGNOSIS

- There are different ways to trigger an upgoing toe response, which along with fanning of the other toes indicates a pyramidal lesion.
- The classical way is to scratch the plantar aspect of the sole by a rough object starting from the lateral side and making an "L" sign as you get closer to the tarsals (Babinski sign).
- If the sole is ulcerated or wrapped, one can scratch the skin close to the lateral malleolus dorsally and get the same effect (Chaddock sign).
- If the foot provides no access to perform either, then a painful sliding pressure over the shin (tibia) will have the same effect (Oppenheim sign).
- It is a good practice to strike the sole when sensory impairment of the feet is accompanied by brisk or even preserved ankle reflexes. In that case, a positive Babinski sign would indicate myelopathy or even encephalopathy as an explanation for the sensory deficit.

SKIN SIGNS

CASE 27.1: CIDP WITH HYPOGONADISM

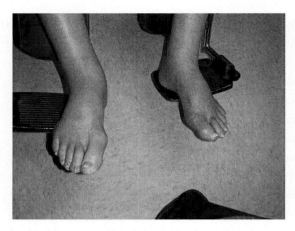

VIDEO 27.1

A 52-year-old man with refractory chronic inflammatory demyelinating polyneuropathy (CIDP) had developed recurrent severe ascites. Computed tomography (CT) abdomen revealed splenomegaly. He also developed hypogonadism, which required testosterone replacement. Gradually he developed the shown skin lesions. Immuno-fixation protein electrophoresis (IFPE) showed immunoglobin A (IgA) monoclonal gammopathy.

The elevation of the following factor in the serum would confirm the diagnosis:

1. Nerve growth factor (NGF)
2. Vascular endothelial growth factor (VEGF)
3. Hepatocyte growth factor (HGF)
4. Brain derived growth factor (BGF)
5. Human chorionic gonadotropin (hCG)

DIAGNOSIS

- Polyneuropathy is the most common manifestation of POEMS syndrome.
- Cutaneous manifestations of POEMS are diverse and none is pathognomonic. They include:
  - Hemangiomas
  - Hyperpigmentation (the most common skin feature)
  - Skin thickening
  - Acrocyanosis
  - Hypertrichosis (associated with endocrine disorders)
  - Facial lipodystrophy
  - Leukonychia
  - Livedo reticularis
- Vascular endothelial growth factor (VEGF) plays an important role in the pathogenesis of POEMS but its role in the genesis of the skin lesions is less clear and its level is not significantly different in patients with skin lesions than in those without.
- Patients with refractory chronic inflammatory demyelinating polyneuropathy (CIDP) should be watched for skin lesions and organomegaly and VEGF should be checked. VEGF is very sensitive but not specific. In POEMS, levels are often very high.
- Peripheral edema, ascites, and pleural effusion are common and carry a bad prognosis.
- Serum M-Protein is present in 85% of cases and therefore, its absence does not exclude POEMS.
- The paraprotein of POEMS syndrome are typically IgG or IgA with lambda light chains, but IgM may occur as well.
- Mild elevation of VEGF occurs in inflammatory neuropathies.
- VEGF is increased early in scleroderma.

REFERENCES

Barete S, et al. Skin manifestations and vascular endothelial growth factor levels in POEMS syndrome: impact of autologous hematopoietic stem cell transplantation. *Arch Dermatol.* 2010;146(6):615–623.

Dispenzieri A, et al. POEMS syndrome: update on diagnosis, risk stratification, and management. *Am J Hematol.* 2012 Aug;87(8):804–814.

CASE 27.2: SKIN RASH AND WEIGHT LOSS

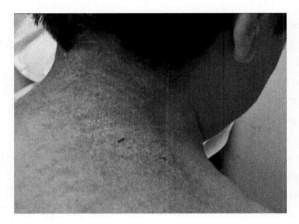

VIDEO 27.2

A 54-year-old woman had developed weight loss and dysphagia over 6 weeks. The mentioned symptoms and signs are consistent with:

1. Scleroderma
2. Systemic lupus erythematosus (SLE)
3. Dermatomyositis (DM)
4. Psoriasis
5. Polymyositis (PM)

DIAGNOSIS

- Cutaneous manifestations of dermatomyositis are diverse.
- Skin lesions are not required for the diagnosis of dermatomyositis (DM), which has characteristic muscle pathology.
- Skin lesions precede myopathy in most cases, and they may never be accompanied by myopathic changes (amyopathic dermatomyositis [DM]).
- Skin eruption of DM is usually itchy and scaly.
- Common skin signs are:
  - Heliotropes and lilac discoloration of the eyelids with periorbital swelling
  - Gottron papules are very characteristic
  - Malar erythema
  - Poikiloderma
  - Photosensitivity
  - Violaceous erythema
  - Periungual telangiectasia
  - Macular rash in the face, upper trunk, anterior neck (V sign), back and shoulders (shawl sign) knees, elbows, neck
  - Thickening and hyperpigmentation are common in chronic cases
  - In dark skin, diagnosis of skin rash may be delayed
- It is important that patients with proximal weakness and or elevated creatinine kinase (CK) are examined for skin lesions and their nail beds are examined with a magnifying lens such as an ophthalmoscopic lens.
- In severe cases, skin lesions coalesce and cover a wide surface area and become very erythematous and itchy. Bullous eruption is also reported.
- Skin lesions usually resolve along the myopathic features with treatment.
- In this case, the knuckle skin, which is typically affected in dermatomyositis, is spared and the rash mostly appeared in the upper back.
- Skin biopsy usually shows chronic inflammatory changes.

CASE 27.3: PUFFY EYES AND SKIN RASH

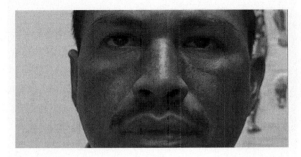

VIDEO 27.3

A 33-year-old man presented with an 8-month history of puffiness around the eyes and rash around the elbows and knees, followed by difficulty climbing stairs. Electromyogram (EMG) was myopathic and creatine phosphokinase (CPK) level was 670 U/L.

The muscle biopsy in this case will likely show:

1. Endomysial inflammation
2. Non-inflammatory myopathy
3. Perifascicular atrophy
4. Cytoplasmic inclusion bodies
5. Red-rimmed vacuoles

Dermatomyositis (Figure 27.3.1):

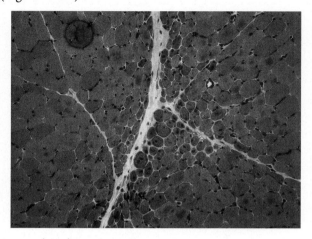

FIGURE 27.3.1 H & E stain (100x): perifascicular atrophy.

DIAGNOSIS

- The pathology shows perifascicular atrophy.
- There is erythematous violaceous rash affecting the knuckles, forehead, and malar areas of the face. This is typically seen in dermatomyositis.
- Pathological changes in dermatomyositis are very characteristic and can be used to make the diagnosis of dermatomyositis even in the absence of skin rash.
- These changes reflect the vascular nature of the disease as opposed to the actual myopathic nature of polymyositis and inclusion body myositis (IBM). The number of the intramuscular blood vessels is reduced.
- The target antigen is located on the intramuscular endothelium and the primary inflammation is perivascular with less prominent invasion of non-necrotic muscle fibers compared to polymyositis (PM).
- The inflammatory infiltrate mainly consists of CD4, confirming the humoral nature of the disease as opposed to the cell-mediated immunity of PM and IBM (increased CD8 count).
- The periphery of the fascicles is the watershed area of these fascicles, and it reflects ischemic changes more than the central areas, leading to atrophy and degeneration of several layers of muscle fibers located on the margin of the fascicles. This feature is called perifascicular atrophy (PFA) and is very highly characteristic of dermatomyositis (DM) but not pathognomonic. PFA also occurs in other vasculopathies like SLE and scleroderma.
- PFA occurs in 60% of cases; therefore, its absence is not against the diagnosis of dermatomyositis.
- Myopathic features such us variation of muscle size and shape, and muscle fiber necrosis and phagocytoses are less pronounced than in PM.
- Increased vacuolation and glycogen contents of some affected fibers are also commonly reported.
- Major histocompatibility complex (MHC) class I expression occurs in 95% of cases.
- Deposition of the membrane attack complex of the intramuscular microvasculature differentiate dermatomyositis from polymyositis and IBM.

CASE 27.4: FOOT ULCER

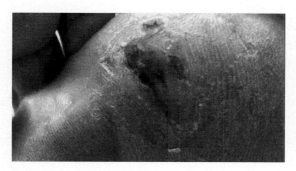

VIDEO 27.4

A patient presented with poorly controlled diabetes mellitus type 2 (DM2) for 20 years. She has neuropathy and peripheral vascular disease (PVD).

The following factors contributed to this ulcer:

1. Neuropathy
2. Peripheral vascular disease
3. Callus formation
4. Trauma
5. Hyperglycemia

DIAGNOSIS

- 50% of diabetics develop foot ulcer sometime during lifetime.
- Diabetic foot is the major cause of hospitalization among diabetics.
- Every year, 85,000 limb amputations occur due to diabetes in the United States.
- Untreated foot ulcer leads to amputation in 85% of cases.
- The skin over the metatarsal heads is vulnerable to pressure due to lack of subcutaneous fat.
- Repeated pressure leads to callus formation, an area with poor circulation that often ulcerates.
- Lack of pain due to neuropathy, poor circulation due to peripheral vascular disease (PVD), and hyperglycemia, which is a favorable media for bacteria to flourish, all contribute to the appearance and progression of a diabetic foot ulcer.
- Minor trauma may cause significant tissue destruction with little pain.
- Osteomyelitis is a common complication.
- Tissue infection spreads quickly and may be life-threatening.
- A non-responsive ulcer to therapy should be debrided, the foot should be rested, and intravenous (IV) antibiotics are administered.
- Special wide shoes are helpful.
- Educated patients who inspect their feet every night are less likely to develop diabetic foot ulcers.

CASE 27.5: SKIN RASH AND NEUROPATHY

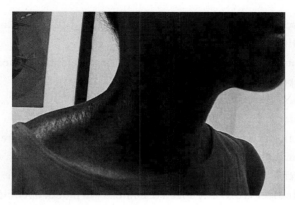

VIDEO 27.5

A 31-year-old woman presented with a 3-year history of dysphagia and skin rash. She then developed severe proximal arm, leg, and neck extensors weakness. Creatinine kinase (CK) level was 250 U/L. Electromyography (EMG) revealed findings of non-irritative myopathy. Nerve conduction study (NCS) revealed evidence of axonal neuropathy. She had been on cyclophosphamide and prednisone for a year when this examination was done. Muscle biopsy revealed endomysial inflammatory changes.

The following occurs in scleroderma but not in dermatomyositis:

1. Proximal weakness
2. Skin rash
3. Dysphagia
4. Neuropathy
5. Progressive course

DIAGNOSIS

- Patients with scleroderma present to the neuromuscular clinic due to skin rash and muscle weakness, thus mimicking dermatomyositis.
- This serious autoimmune illness has a spectrum of presentations; the most serious is progressive widespread sclerosis of the skin and internal organs.
- Raynaud phenomenon is common.
- It targets females at age 30–50 years.
- Skin lesions: the skin is thick, shiny, and adherent. It is different from the violaceous erythematous rash and periorbital discoloration and edema that are typical for dermatomyositis.
- Arms, trunk, and face are mostly affected. Difficulty in mouth opening and contracture of extremities is a typical feature.
- Gastrointestinal (dysphagia, diarrhea), cardiac (pericarditis), and pulmonary (fibrosis) involvement is common.
- Neuropathies are common in scleroderma but are not a feature of dermatomyositis and they include:
  - Trigeminal neuropathy
  - Asymmetric painful sensorimotor axonal neuropathy (vasculitic)
  - Entrapment neuropathies
- Polymyositis (overlap syndrome) is not uncommon. Polymyositis-scleroderma (PM-Scl) antibodies are usually positive.
- Vascular endothelial growth factor (VEGF) level is increased.

REFERENCES

http://neuromuscular.wustl.edu

Ringel RA, et al. Muscle involvement in the scleroderma syndrome. *Arch Intern Med.* 1990 Dec;150(12): 2550–2552.

CASE 27.6: HARD SKIN IN A UREMIC PATIENT

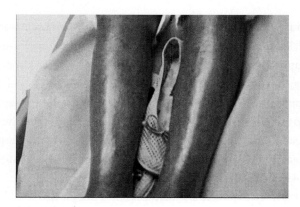

VIDEO 27.6

A 70-year-old woman on hemodialysis for 5 years had an MRI of the neck for radicular symptoms. Two weeks after the MRI, she developed pain and stiffness of the legs, and she could not walk any more. Her skin was very tight and firm and was attached to the underlying structures.

The most likely diagnosis is:

1. Scleroderma
2. Systemic sclerosis
3. Dermatomyositis
4. Nephrogenic systemic fibrosis (NSF)
5. Systemic lupus erythematosus (SLE)

DIAGNOSIS

- These patients are referred to neuromuscular clinics due to muscle weakness and hardening of the skin, leading to suspicion of scleroderma or dermatomyositis.
- Nephrogenic systemic fibrosis (NSF) is due to fibrosis of the skin and other structures like heart, lung, and muscle in hemodialysis patients who receive gadolinium.
  - 5% of patients with renal impairment who received gadolinium developed NSF.
- Excessive exposure of renal patients to gadolinium is damaging to the tissue.
- Avoidance of gadolinium in high-risk patients leads to a dramatic drop in reported cases.
- Pathological features are due to proliferation of fibrocyte and histiocytes and collagen bundles. CD34+ dermal dendrites are abundant.
- Latent period between exposure and disease is 2–4 weeks.
- Typical lesions are focal, edematous, and tender and turn into hard confluent lesions in the legs and arms, then the chest and abdomen, while sparing the head.
- Muscle fibrosis, confirmed by MRI and biopsy, is reported with minimal weakness and significant joint contracture.
- Sed rate and eosinophil count are usually high, but CK is usually normal. EMG is myopathic or shows decreased insertional activity due to fibrosis.
- The disease is progressive, but 40% of cases go into remission after the dialysis is stopped.
- Gadolinium should be avoided when glomerular filtration rate (GFR) is less than 50 ml/min.
- Renal transplantation is the best hope. Plasma exchange (PLEX) is reported to be beneficial.

REFERENCE

Levine JM, et al. Involvement of skeletal muscle in dialysis-associated systemic fibrosis (nephrogenic fibrosing dermopathy). *Muscle Nerve.* 2004;30(5):569.

CASE 27.7: POLYMYOSITIS AND EAR EROSION

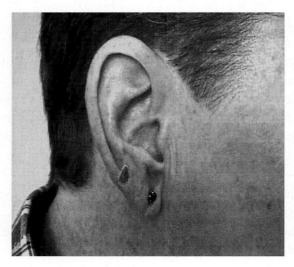

VIDEO 27.7

A 65-year-old woman presented with history of polymyositis (PM) with bilateral ear pain and trachitis.

These lesions are typically seen in:

1. Relapsing polychondritis
2. Scleroderma
3. Vasculitis
4. POEMS (polyneuropathy, organomegaly, endocrinopathy, monoclonal gammopathy, and skin changes)
5. Nephrogenic systemic fibrosis

DIAGNOSIS

- Relapsing polychondritis (RPC) is an autoimmune inflammation of the cartilaginous structures (ears, nose, joints, eyes, respiratory tract).
- At least one-third of the cases are associated with systemic inflammatory conditions such as vasculitis and polymyositis.
- Auricular involvement is the most common feature, and it is the presenting finding in 40% of cases.
- Recurrent attacks lead to deformity of the ears and nose (saddle nose).
- Hoarseness, aphonia, stridor, dyspnea, and cough indicate respiratory tract involvement.
- Polyarthritis, heart valvular disease, renal involvement, gastrointestinal (GI), and skin involvement are usual.
- Encephalopathy (seizures, hemiplegia, dementia), myelopathy, and inflammatory neuropathy are well reported.
- Different types of systemic vasculitis occur in 25% of cases and are associated with poor prognosis.
- Other autoimmune diseases such as Graves disease, rheumatoid arthritis (RA), SLE, ulcerative colitis, and polymyositis are reported.
- There are no specific serological markers or pathological findings for this condition. The diagnosis is made mostly based on the inflammation of multiple cartilaginous structures.
- The disease is generally responsive to steroids and steroid-sparing agents but is occasionally fatal, and most of the time recurrent attacks lead to cumulative disability.
- Neuromuscular patients with cough, wheezes, progressive neuropathy, and/or myopathy and hematuria should be investigated for RPC as well as other possibilities such as Wagner granulomatosis and Sturge Strauss disease.

CASE 27.8: DILATED CAPILLARIES AND PROXIMAL WEAKNESS

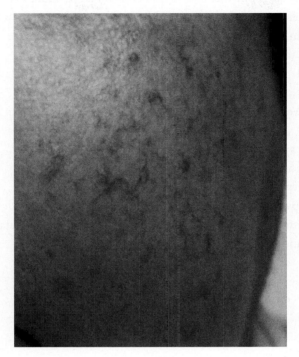

VIDEO 27.8

A 62-year-old woman presented with scleroderma w.th proximal weakness and skin lesions. These skin lesions are:

1. Telangiectasias
2. Varicose veins
3. Spider Nevi
4. Hemangiomas
5. None of the above

DIAGNOSIS

- Telangiectasia means small dilated loops of blood vessels, usually capillaries.
- It usually develops in the face, legs, and less commonly in other parts of the body.
- It may occur in normal people due to sun skin damage and aging.
- Neurological and neuromuscular associations:
  - Congenital:
    - Ataxia telangiectasia
    - Sturge-Weber syndrome
  - Acquired:
    - Cushing syndrome including chronic steroid therapy
    - Carcinoid syndrome
    - Scleroderma
- LASER therapy and sclerotherapy are usually effective.
- The most common two causes of proximal weakness and telangiectasia are chronic steroid therapy and scleroderma.

CASE 27.9: PROXIMAL WEAKNESS, ASTHMA, AND SKIN RASH

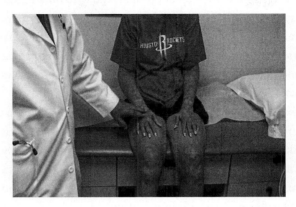

VIDEO 27.9

A 50-year-old woman presented with weight loss, bronchial asthma, muscle weakness, and skin rash that had evolved over a few months. CPK level was 450 U/L. Peripheral eosinophil count was 34%. EMG revealed findings of irritative myopathy and axonal polyneuropathy. ESR was 87 mm/hr. Nerve biopsy is shown (Figure 27.9.1).

The most likely diagnosis is:

1. Dermatomyositis
2. Systemic lupus erythematosus (SLE)
3. Vasculitis
4. Scleroderma
5. POEMS (polyneuropathy, organomegaly, endocrinopathy, monoclonal gammopathy, and skin changes)

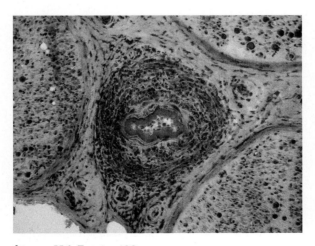

FIGURE 27.9.1 Nerve biopsy; H & E stain: 400x.

DIAGNOSIS

- Nerve biopsy image shows invasion of vascular wall with inflammatory cells.
- Progressive asymmetrical axonal painful neuropathy and erythematous and purpuric skin rash are very suggestive of vasculitis. Proximal weakness suggests myositis; high ESR and CK levels support the diagnosis of vasculitis, which is confirmed by nerve biopsy.
- Skin rash is one of the important manifestations of systemic vasculitis, and it is due to inflammation of the cutaneous blood vessels.
- Cutaneous vasculitis may be the only feature of vasculitis, although more frequently it is part of a systemic picture with involvement of the peripheral nervous system (PNS).
- Pathology of skin lesions does not always reflect the picture of the systemic vasculitis; as an example, it may not show granuloma in Wegner or Churg-Struass vasculitis. Therefore, skin biopsy is usually not adequate for the diagnosis and a muscle and/or nerve biopsy are more likely to provide more specific information.
- Skin lesions usually show fibrinoid necrosis and perivascular neurotrophilic infiltration.
- Palpable purpura:
  - Is very characteristic of cutaneous vasculitis.
  - Maculopapular rash usually precedes palpable purpura.
  - These purpuras do not blanch by pressure, unlike simple purpura.
  - They are caused by extravasation of erythrocytes through damaged blood vessels.
  - They are more common in the legs and buttocks because the increased hydrostatic pressure predisposes the body to their formation.
  - Purpura has many other causes, such as thromboembolism due to hyperviscosity, malignancy, and so on.
  - Antiphospholipid syndrome may produce purpura that can be confused with vasculitis, but the former usually is associated with livedo reticularis in the legs.
- Cutaneous vasculitis may affect the scalp, causing alopecia.
- Exacerbation of the skin lesions usually correlates with the exacerbation of systemic vasculitis and they heal together.

CASE 27.10: INSENSITIVE FEET TO ANT BITES

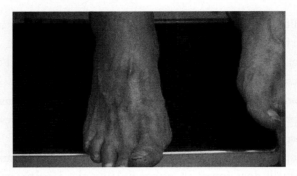

VIDEO 27.10

A 50-year-old diabetic patient noticed red spots on his feet every time he worked in the back-yard. Some of these lesions became infected. He had no foot pain. Examination is shown. During examination, he was found to have a lesion on the left forehead, and he gave a history of seizures.

The following is (are) true regarding the feet lesions:

1. They are likely a manifestation of diabetic neuropathy.
2. They are related to the port wine stain on the forehead.
3. They may lead to gangrene and amputation.
4. They are vascular in nature.
5. This is a normal response to a specific kind of ants.

DIAGNOSIS

- Diabetes mellitus (DM) is the most common cause of neuropathy in the United States (leprosy is the first internationally).
- Diabetic vascular and neuropathic complications are the most common cause of non-traumatic amputations.
- Diabetes is associated with 10 types of neuropathies, the most common of which is distal symmetrical predominantly sensory polyneuropathy, which evolves gradually and may precede the diagnosis of DM by up to 2 years.
- Sensory neuropathy may present with pain, but more so, it presents with numbness of the feet that usually does not get attention until unnoticed injuries, such as shoe-induced trauma or insect bites, occur repeatedly.
- These skin lesions are vulnerable to spreading infection due to the associated hyperglycemia and vascular insufficiency, and they may lead to gangrene.
- Diabetics should always be instructed to inspect their feet every night for skin lesions.
- The left forehead lesion is a port wine stain. This birthmark may occur anywhere on the skin and is usually an isolated and benign condition.
- Port wine stain may be associated with cerebral vascular abnormalities (Sturge Weber syndrome), leading to seizures.
- Neuropathy is not a feature of Sturge Weber syndrome but may be a feature of other phacomatoses (neurocutaneous syndromes), such as neurofibromatosis.
- Phacomatoses are disorders of the CNS, skin, and sometimes eye due to shared ectodermal origin of these structures and include:
  1. Neurofibromatosis
  2. Tuberous sclerosis
  3. Ataxia telangiectasia
  4. Sturge-Weber syndrome
  5. von Hippel-Lindau disease
  6. Incontinentia pigmenti
  7. Nevoid basal cell carcinoma syndrome
  8. Wyburn-Mason syndrome

CHAPTER 28

EMG FINDINGS

CASE 28.1: DYSARTHRIA AND PARASPINAL SPONTANEOUS ACTIVITY

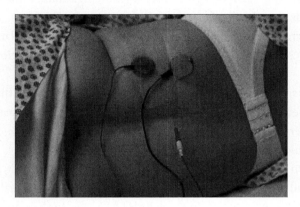

VIDEO 28.1

A 65-year-old woman presented with a seven-month history of slurring of speech and swallowing difficulty. She noticed heaviness and twitching of the arms. Creatine kinase (CK) level was 530 IU/ml. Among other findings, the thoracic paraspinal muscles and tongue showed the demonstrated activity.

These discharges are:

1. Specific for amyotrophic lateral sclerosis
2. Specific for inflammatory myopathies
3. Irregular
4. Not visible by physical examination
5. Single fiber EMG (SFEMG) of an affected muscle may show an increased jitter

DIAGNOSIS

- Fibrillations are spontaneous regular discharges of single muscle fibers, and they are typically seen in denervation but also seen in inflammatory myopathies.
- Fibrillations are not visible by physical examination, unlike fasciculations.
- The initial positivity (negative deflection) differentiates fibrillations from end plate potentials.
- Thoracic paraspinal muscles are very sensitive for fibrillations and they should be tested routinely, especially if motor neuron disease or inflammatory myopathies are suspected. They are preferred over lumbar and cervical paraspinal muscles, which are common targets for radiculopathies.
- It may take up to 2 weeks for fibrillations to appear after an insult, depending on how far the affected muscle is from the injured nerve. Thoracic paraspinal muscles (TPS) are affected early in amyotrophic lateral sclerosis (ALS) due to their proximity to the motor neurons and therefore El Escorial criteria count the thoracic regions as one of four important regions (cervical, lumbar, and bulbar) where denervation should be looked for in ALS suspects.
- Fibrillations do not resolve immediately after the cause is treated, and they may stay for years or permanently. Often fibrillation potentials from a long-standing injury become very low amplitude. Therefore, paraspinal muscles in a surgically treated lumbar or cervical spines lose their value as indicators of new denervation, although some studies suggest that if you see a large amplitude fibrillation potentials in the lumbar paraspinal muscles in a patient with prior lumbar surgery, it may reflect more recent denervation.
- Single fiber EMG (SFEMG) is a very sensitive test for myasthenia gravis (MG). A negative test in a weak muscle excludes MG.
- SFEMG is not specific and is positive in early re-innervation due to remodeling of the motor unit. Such changes can be seen in motor neuron disease, polyneuropathies, radiculopathies, and polymyositis.

CASE 28.2: LEG PAIN AND SPONTANEOUS FAST ACTIVITY

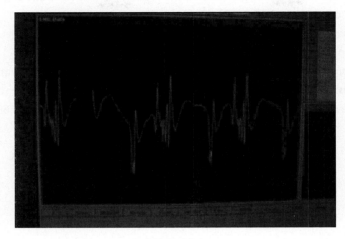

VIDEO 28.2

A 72-year-old-woman presented with chronic lower back pain radiating to the right calf and numbness of the lateral aspect of the right foot. She had absent right ankle reflex and history of L5 laminectomy seven years earlier with pain relief for a year. Electromyography (EMG) showed the demonstrated finding in the right gastrocnemius.

These discharges are:

1. Specific for myopathy
2. Specific for radiculopathy
3. Specific for chronic denervation
4. Specific for amyotrophic lateral sclerosis (ALS)
5. Nonspecific

DIAGNOSIS

- Complex repetitive discharges (CRDs) are regular spontaneous discharges of groups of muscle fibers that occur in non rhythmic bursts.
- The fibers are activated ephaptically.
- Usual firing rate is 30–40 Hz.
- Abrupt onset and end differentiate them from the waxing and waning myotonic discharges.
- CRDs are not specific and occur in chronic neurogenic and myopathic conditions.

CASE 28.3: SKIN RASH AND SHORT DURATION UNITS

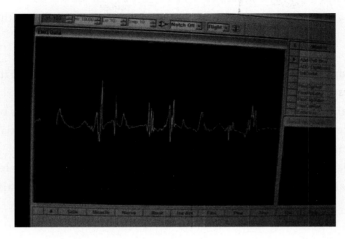

VIDEO 28.3

A 36-year-old woman presented with a 6-month history of difficulty climbing stairs and fatigue. She had symmetrical proximal weakness of the legs and arms and a CK level of 800 IU/L. Skin lesions are shown.

The mentioned findings suggest:

1. Dermatomyositis
2. Polymyositis
3. Amyotrophic lateral sclerosis (ALS)
4. Inclusion body myositis (IBM)
5. Systemic lupus erythematosus (SLE)

DIAGNOSIS

Electromyography (EMG) in myopathies:

Electromyography (EMG) is a useful tool to diagnose myopathies with the following limitations:

- Some myopathies do not usually cause EMG abnormalities except late in the course of the disease, such as mitochondrial and metabolic myopathies.
- A well-trained operator is needed in order to detect the subtle changes of some myopathies since low amplitude very brief short duration motor unit potentials interspersed with normal motor unit potentials are hard to detect.
- In chronic myopathies, mixed short and long duration potentials may lead to diagnostic confusion. Observing the recruitment rate of motor unit potentials can help sort this out.

The following findings are seen in myopathies:
- Short duration, low amplitude, polyphasic units with early recruitment. Proximal muscles are the first to demonstrate such units in most myopathies.
- Spontaneous discharges (fibrillation and sharp waves) especially in thoracic paraspinal muscles are commonly seen in inflammatory, metabolic, and toxic myopathies. Irritative myopathy is commonly used to describe myopathies with spontaneous discharges.

The proximal weakness, skin rash, elevated CK level, and irritative myopathic findings in the demonstrated case was very consistent with dermatomyositis.

CASE 28.4: FAMILIAL NEUROGENIC FIRING

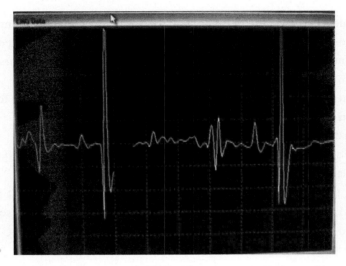

VIDEO 28.4

A 40-year-old Hispanic man presented with a 20-year history of dysarthria and muscle twitching. He had a brother with the same problems. He had tongue fasciculations and diffuse areflexia with mild sensory impairment in the feet. CK level was 1,300 IU/L. The shown finding was seen in all the tested muscles in the arms and legs.

He most likely has:

1. Androgen receptor mutation (AR mutation)
2. Superoxide dismutase mutation (SOD mutation)
3. Polymyositis
4. Sporadic amyotrophic lateral sclerosis (ALS)
5. TAR DNA-binding protein 43 Mutation (TDP43 mutation)

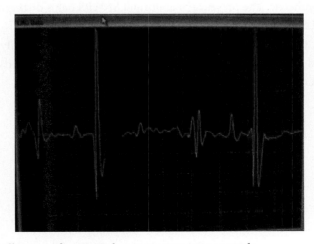

FIGURE 28.4.1 A still screen of an EMG showing motor unit potentials.

DIAGNOSIS

- Chronic denervation is usually associated with re-innervation. The re-innervated motor units produce high amplitude (20 millivolt in this case; NL: 4) and long duration potentials (normal 5–15 msec.). Due to loss of synchrony, polyphasicity occurs (normal value is up to three phases).

- The frequency of firing of motor units increases in order to compensate for the neuronal loss; therefore this finding is one of the hallmarks of denervation.

- There are different ways to calculate firing frequency:
  - ◆ Set the sweep at 1,000 and count the number of times that a specific single motor unit potential appears in the screen at the time a second unit starts firing.
  - ◆ Count the number of seconds between two identical motor unit potentials and divide 1,000 (milliseconds) by that number. In this case there are 5 squares between the two units (50 milliseconds) and therefore the firing frequency (FF) is 20 Hz (Normal: 10) (Figure 28.4.1).

- "Recruitment pattern" is a term used to measure the amount of units recruited with maximum contraction. If there are not enough units to fill the screen, recruitment is said to be decreased. Due to potential for muscle injury and pain during contraction, this method is obsolete.

- There are occasions when recruitment is decreased but firing frequency is normal. This is typically seen in central causes such as stroke, myelopathy, and hysterical weakness or poor effort. When the problem is of a lower motor neuron nature, fast firing of normal appearing motor unit potentials can also be an important clue that muscle weakness is caused by a demyelinating process, due to a partial conduction block proximally.

- Kennedy disease is a chronic hereditary lower motor neuron disease that affects both bulbar and spinal muscles. Electromyography (EMG) is very important to reveal the chronic widespread chronic denervation and to rule out myopathy that is suspected due to elevated CK level that is common in this disease. The very stable chronic appearing motor unit potentials with fairly symmetric findings helps differentiate Kennedy disease from ALS, where motor unit potentials are usually very polyphasic and unstable and (initially at least) asymmetric. The presence of abnormal SNAPS helps distinguish Kennedy disease from ALS and the spinal muscular atrophies.

- In this case, the chronic diffusely denervating process with a family history, elevated CK level, and abnormal sensory responses strongly suggested Kennedy disease, which is caused by mutation of androgen receptors gene.

CASE 28.5: SPONTANEOUS ACTIVITY AFTER RADIOTHERAPY

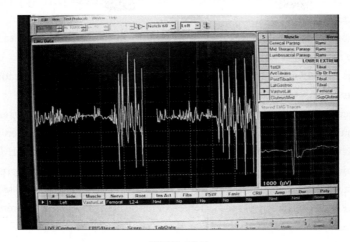

VIDEO 28.5

A 65-year-old woman with a history of rectal cancer 8 years earlier presented with progressive asymmetrical painless leg weakness. She had normal sensation and absent knee reflexes and normal sural responses. The demonstrated activity is obtained from the right thigh adductors.

These findings represent:

1. Myokymia
2. Myotonia
3. Neuromyotonia
4. Complex repetitive discharges
5. Artifacts

DIAGNOSIS

- Radiation is toxic to the motor neurons, and the neurotoxic effect may not appear until several years after the exposure.
- Slowly progressive painless weakness and atrophy in the regions distal to the irradiated area is the first symptom.
- Symptoms may progress for a few months and then plateau. The exact cause is not clear. Vascular injury and DNA repair malfunction have been proposed.
- Recurrence of the tumor is typically associated with more pain and progressive course.
- Myokymia is highly characteristic of this syndrome but can also be seen in focal nerve injury such as multifocal motor neuropathy with conduction block (MMNCB), carpal tunnel syndrome (CTS), brainstem glioma, and multiple sclerosis. The presence of myokymia in a weak limb that had prior radiation treatment for cancer very strongly suggests that the weakness is from post-radiation changes rather than from recurrent tumor, especially if the weakness is painless.
- Myokymia is a rhythmic spontaneous discharge of the same motor unit and is repeated every 0.1–3/sec (of bursts)
- Frequency of the potentials is 5–70 Hz. Each burst may have 2–7 potentials.

CASE 28.6: CHRONIC FAMILIAL WEAKNESS

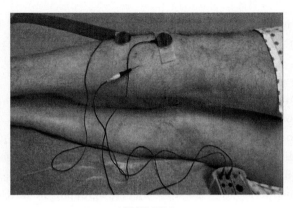

VIDEO 28.6

A 51-year-old man presented with chronic weakness and atrophy of the bilateral distal leg muscles and areflexia. His mother had similar symptoms

The shown discharges:

1. Have high amplitude
2. Have a firing rate below 10HZ
3. Indicate chronic denervation
4. Are myopathic
5. Indicate acute denervation

DIAGNOSIS

- The recorded motor unit potentials have an amplitude of 10 mV (gain is 1,000 mV) and firing frequency of 25Hz. These are re-innervated large units and indicate chronic denervation.
- Chronic denervation with normal sensory responses suggest:
  1. Radiculopathy
  2. Motor neuron disease
  3. Rarely, motor neuropathy
- Chronic and diffuse denervation with positive family history suggests chronic familial motor neuron disease such as spinal muscular atrophy.
- Re-innervation units are responsible for fiber type grouping in muscle biopsy.

CASE 28.7: DECELERATING MOTORCYCLE ENGINE

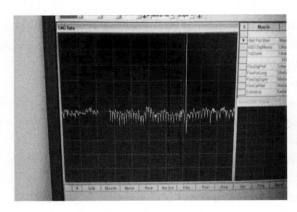

VIDEO 28.7

A 55-year-old woman presented with muscle stiffness for several years. Her father had a premature Christmas tree cataract. The patient has a pacemaker.

The following mutation is responsible for this condition:

1. Cytosine-thymine-guanine (CTG) repeat expansion
2. CTG repeat contraction
3. A mutation in the coding region of the dystrophia myotonica-protein kinase (DMPK) gene
4. Stable mutation
5. Autosomal recessive gene

DIAGNOSIS

- Myotonic discharges are spontaneous muscle fiber discharges noticed by needle EMG.
- They appear, like many fibrillations, as positive sharp waves with waxing and waning frequency and amplitude.
- Firing frequency 20–40 Hz
- Accelerating and decelerating motorcycle engine (in military terms, dive bomber).
- Neuromyotonia: frequency is more than 150 Hz and complex repetitive discharges (CRDs) have abrupt onset and outset.
- Myotonic discharges correlate with slow muscle relaxation clinically.
- They occur in myotonic disorders, dystrophic and non-dystrophic, and in metabolic, toxic, and inflammatory myopathies.
- They are more prominent in distal muscles.
- CTG repeat expansion correlates with severity and age of onset but it is not clear if it is correlated with the severity of electrical myotonia, which varies from one muscle to another.
- CTG repeat expansion varies among different tissue but not among different muscles, despite variability in strength.

SUPPLEMENT FOR THE CASE 15.8

Classification and diagnostic criteria for inclusion body myositis (IBM):

I. Characteristic Features: Inclusion Criteria
    A. Clinical features
        - Duration of illness: greater than 6 months
        - Age of onset: greater than 30 years old
        - Muscle weakness
            - Must affect proximal and distal muscles of arms and legs and
            - Patient must exhibit at least one of the following features:
                - Finger flexor weakness
                - Wrist flexor greater than wrist extensor weakness
                - Quadriceps muscle weakness (equal to or less than grade 4 MRC)
    B. Laboratory features
        - Serum creatine kinase less than 12 times normal
        - Muscle biopsy
            - Inflammatory myopathy characterized by mononuclear cell invasion of non-necrotic muscle fibers
            - Vacuolated muscle fibers
            - Either:
                - Intracellular amyloid deposits (must use fluorescent method of identification before excluding the presence of amyloid) or 15–18-nm tubulofilaments by electron microscopy
        - Electromyography must be consistent with features of inflammatory myopathy (however, long duration potentials are commonly observed and do not exclude diagnosis of sporadic inclusion body myositis)

II. Diagnostic criteria for inclusion body myositis
    A. Definite inclusion body myositis
        - Patient must exhibit all muscle biopsy features, including invasion of non-necrotic fibers by mononuclear cells, vacuolated muscle fibers, and intracellular (within muscle fibers) amyloid deposits or 15–18-nm tubulofilaments
        - None of the other clinical or laboratory features is mandatory if muscle biopsy features are diagnostic
    B. Possible inclusion body myositis
        - If the muscle biopsy shows only inflammation (invasion of non-necrotic muscle fibers by mononuclear cells) without other pathological features of inclusion body myositis, then a diagnosis of possible inclusion body myositis can be given if the patient exhibits the characteristic clinical and laboratory features

INDEX